INTERMITTENT FASTING FOR WOMEN OVER 50

THE NEW STEP-BY-STEP GUIDE TO LOSE WEIGHT FAST WITHOUT HUNGER PANGS. THE BEST WAY TO ENJOY INTERMITTENT FASTING WITH DELICIOUS RECIPES TO RESET METABOLISM

Written By
Natalie Olsson

Table of Contents

Introduction

What Is Intermittent Fasting?

Intermittent fasting is a form of weight loss diet that limits your calorie intake for days, weeks, or months at a time and then allows you to eat however much you want on the other days. It's often considered easier than traditional diets because no counting calories, or worrying about "good" and "bad" foods is required. There are many variations of intermittent fasting, but the most common type involves only eating during a certain window. This means that when you're not hungry or feeling deprived and tiredness hits it's time to eat again!

The basis of intermittent fasting is that the body isn't constantly digesting food and thus more energy is available for fat loss. This technique can therefore be used as a way to lose weight and keep it off!

Intermittent fasting (IF) is an umbrella term for various calorie restriction patterns in which you cycle between periods of eating and fasting. It's been around for centuries (both religious figures and the Buddha have promoted it), but only recently has there been scientific interest.

There are different intermittent fasting protocols. Some are stuck in the low-carb realm, some have switched to high-carb, and others still (like myself) get both right. But they all share one thing. They make you automatically burn more fat during the fasting periods because of the hormones they affect.

While it is a good idea to adopt an eating schedule that promotes weight loss, it is also important not to fast for too long. Fasting for a few days or weeks should not be harmful, but multiple days of fasting may result in health issues as well as metabolic instability and can lead to unhealthy conditions such as heart failure and diabetes.

What's the Reason for Fasting?

Our body has an innate ability to regulate our blood glucose levels by regulating the release of insulin and glucagon. The hormones that control our response to food and our body's energy production (glucose and fats) are secreted by the pancreatic islets of Langerhans.

These islets release the hormones secretin, gastrin, cholecystokinin, GLP-1, and PYY. All these endocrine controls are intricately connected; for example, when we eat food that contains protein, our pancreas releases insulin, which triggers hormone secretion in the gut. When we eat food that contains fat, our pancreas releases glucagon, which triggers hormone secretion in the gut. This release of hormones causes the release of glucose into the bloodstream and stimulates the liver to process it into glycogen.

How IF Works?

Did you know that skipping a meal can help you lose weight faster? That's right; if you want to slim down a little bit faster, then it's time to start intermittent fasting. But how does it work?

Intermittent fasting isn't really an eating plan; it's primarily an exercise in behavioral shifts. The idea is that by extending the length of time between certain meals—typically breakfast and lunch—to 12 to 14 hours, your body thinks it's been either starved or abandoned and starts to burn fat as its primary fuel source instead of carbohydrates. The end result is massively improved insulin sensitivity and blood sugar regulation paired with increased weight loss.

Does that mean you've got to starve yourself every day? Not at all, but it does mean that you have to rethink your relationship with food. If you're still doing the three big things wrong, intermittent fasting is exactly what you need.

What's Wrong About Intermittent Fasting?

When people think of intermittent fasting, they often think of crazy regimens involving juice fasts or massive amounts of exercise (or both) that are unsustainable and not a lot of fun. That's because most "diets" or "cycles" are built on one thing: deprivation. And deprivation puts your body into survival mode, burning only the bare minimum just to get by.

CHAPTER 1:

The Secret of IF for Women

Because women's bodies were physiologically designed to carry babies, they're more sensitive to potential starvation than men. If a woman's body senses any impending starvation, it will respond by increasing the hormones leptin and ghrelin, which work together to control hunger. This hormonal response is the female body's way of protecting a developing fetus, even if a woman is not currently pregnant.

Although it's possible to ignore the hunger signals from ghrelin and leptin, it becomes increasingly difficult, especially as the body revolts and starts to produce more of these hormones. If a woman gives in to the hunger in an unhealthy way by overeating or consuming unhealthy foods, this can cause a cascade of other hormonal issues involving insulin. This process can also shut down the reproductive system. If your body thinks it doesn't have enough food to survive, it might shut down the ability to conceive to protect a potential pregnancy. This is why fasting is not recommended during pregnancy or for women who are trying to become pregnant.

In women, the release of FSH and LH triggers the ovaries and the production of estrogen and progesterone. The increase in estrogen and progesterone is what causes the release of a mature egg (ovulation). This hormonal cascade usually happens in a regular cycle. However, GnRH is extremely sensitive and can be thrown off by fasting.

It is an open secret that men and women differ in many ways. Some differences are not only physical but emotional and mental between men and women. Consequently, you are not supposed to measure women and men with the same yardstick because it can be problematic.

The main thing that makes it mandatory for us to treat women differently than men is the ability of women to give birth. This is an ability that is only possessed by women. The ability to bear offsprings needs a special body and hormonal structuring. Consequently, you can speak about all the feminism, equality, and any other issue but nothing should go against or underestimate the fact that women have a different hormonal and physical structure that requires special attention.

Physiologically, a woman's body has a higher body fat percentage than men's. While a man may have an ideal essential body fat ratio of 3 to 5 percent, a woman may have it anywhere between 10 to 13 percent. Even in athletes, the male body fat ratio lies between 6 to 13 percent, whereas the female body fat ratio can be as high as 14 to 20 percent. In average body type men, the body fat ratio should fall between 18 to 24 percent. This ratio in women is between 25 to 31 percent.

Effects of Fasting on the Hormonal System of Women

Effect of estrogen imbalance

- Low energy.
- Poor cognitive function.
- Poor heart health.
- Infertility.
- Decreased bone density.
- Poor muscle tone.
- Reduced skin and hair health.
- Poor glucose regulation.
- Gaining unnecessary weight.

Imbalance can also trip the cortisol levels in your body. It is the stress hormone. The impact would be:

- Sugar cravings.
- Fatigue.
- Insomnia.
- Anxiety.
- Low energy.

Thyroid imbalance can also take place. It may lead to:

- Gaining weight.
- Fog in the brain.
- Anxiety.
- Dry hair and dry skin.
- Depression.
- Inconsistent periods.
- The feeling of hot or cold flashes.

Things for Women to Remember While Practicing IF

At some point in your life, you've probably experienced the symptoms of low blood sugar, hunger, irritability, weakness, sweaty palms, or anxiety when you've gone too long without eating. While it's true that low blood sugar can be unpleasant, it's not the fact that you've gone without eating that causes your blood sugar to dip too low: it's what you ate during your previous meal.

When you eat a meal that's loaded with carbohydrates, it sends a rush of glucose into your bloodstream. Your body responds to the glucose rush by releasing insulin to carry it into the cells so you can use it as energy. The higher your glucose spikes, the more insulin that's sent out; the more insulin that's sent out, the more your blood sugar ultimately drops over time. When you combine fasting with a healthy, moderate, low-carbohydrate diet, your body is extremely efficient in managing blood glucose levels on its own so you don't experience those dramatic spikes and dips in your blood sugar even when you go for an extended time without eating.

If you have problems with blood sugar control or if you're diabetic, the glucose and insulin response doesn't work as well, so make sure to speak with your healthcare provider before starting any type of fast to determine if it's right for you.

Eat Mindfully

A meal should be something that you savor, not something that you rush through at your desk while working or in your car between errands. Part of optimal health is eating slowly and mindfully so that you can enjoy every bite, and you can pay attention to signals that tell you when you've had enough. Since you'll be eating fewer meals when you're intermittent fasting, it's even more of a reason to slow down and enjoy the process.

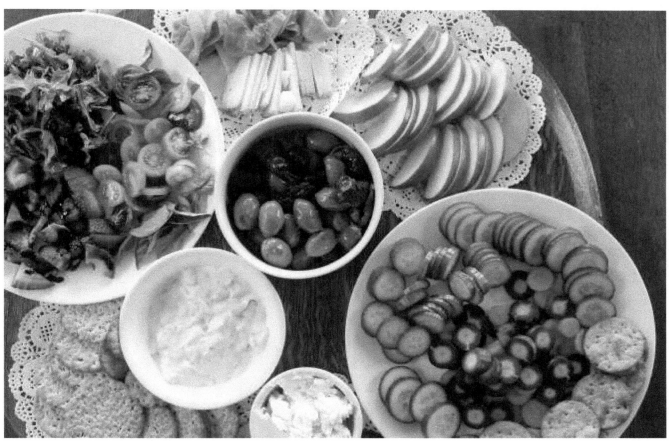

Ingredients for a Healthy Fasting Diet

The intermittent fasting lifestyle is not just about skipping meals; it's also about being more aware of what foods you *do* eat. Just as there are various methods of fasting, there are different diets you can follow, including Paleo, low-carb, and Pegan. You need to find the one that works for you and accomplishes what you want. In addition, you need to make good choices when food shopping, finding foods, and drinks that promote maximum health.

CHAPTER 2:

Top IF Benefits

Intermittent Fasting Affects the Role of Cells, Genes & Hormones

Many things occur in your body when you do not eat for quite a while. For instance, your body begins crucial processes of cellular repair and adjusts the hormone levels so that contained body fat becomes more available. These are some of the changes that take place during the fast in your body:

- **Insulin levels:** insulin levels drop dramatically in the blood, which promotes burning fat.
- **Human growth hormone:** growth hormone blood levels can rise as much as five times as high. Increased levels of this hormone promote burning fat and building muscle and have several other advantages.
- **Cellular repair:** your body causes essential mechanisms of cellular repair, like cell waste removal.
- **Gene expression:** a variety of genes & molecules have beneficial modifications concerning survival and disease prevention.

Intermittent Fasting May Help You Lose Weight as Well as Belly Fat

Most of those who attempt intermittent fasting do so to simply lose weight; intermittent fasting can help you consume fewer meals. If you make up for it by eating even more throughout the various meals, you may end up consuming fewer calories.

Intermittent Fasting May Decrease Insulin Resistance, Reducing Your Possibility of Type 2 Diabetes

In recent decades, type 2 diabetes has now become extremely prevalent. Its key characteristic in terms of insulin resistance is higher blood sugar levels. Anything that increases insulin resistance would help reduce blood sugar levels as well as defend against type 2 diabetes. Curiously, intermittent fasting is shown to have major advantages for insulin resistance, contributing to a remarkable drop in blood sugar.

Intermittent Fasting May Reduce Oxidative Stress & Body Inflammation

One of its moves towards aging, as well as other chronic diseases, is oxidative stress. It includes unstable molecules, known as free radicals that react to and damage other essential molecules (such as protein and DNA). Many studies indicate that intermittent fasting can improve the body's oxidative stress resistance.

Intermittent Fasting Could Be Advantageous for Heart Health

Heart disease is the greatest killer in the world right now. It is understood that specific health indicators ("risk factors") are either associated with an enhanced or reduced risk of heart disease. Numerous specific risk factors like blood pressure, total plus LDL cholesterol, inflammatory markers, and also blood sugar levels have been shown to strengthen by intermittent fasting.

Intermittent Fasting Causes Different Mechanisms for Cellular Repair

The body cells initiate a process of cellular "waste removal" called autophagy when we fast. It includes breaking down the cells and metabolizing the damaged and defective proteins that, over time, build up within the cells. Enhanced autophagy could provide defense against a variety of illnesses, including cancer and Alzheimer's.

Intermittent Fasting Can Help Prevent Cancer

Cancer is a horrible disease that is defined by uncontrolled cell growth. Fasting is shown to have some positive effects on metabolism, which may contribute to reduced cancer risk. Despite the need for human studies, promising indications from animal studies suggests that intermittent fasting can help to prevent cancer.

Intermittent Fasting Is Helpful for Your Brain

Sometimes, what is beneficial to the body is good for the brain too. Intermittent fasting enhances the different metabolic features that are considered to be critical for brain health. It involves lowered oxidative stress, decreased inflammation, and decreased levels of blood sugar as well as insulin resistance. Several rat studies have also shown that intermittent fasting can stimulate the development of new nerve cells, which will improve brain function.

Intermittent Fasting Can Help With Alzheimer's Disease Prevention

Alzheimer's disease is the most prevalent neurodegenerative illness in the world. There is no treatment available regarding Alzheimer's, and it is important to prevent it from occurring. A rat study shows intermittent fasting can postpone the emergence of Alzheimer's disease or decrease its severity. Animal studies also show that fasting will defend against all other neurodegenerative disorders, including diseases caused by Parkinson's & Huntington's. There is still a need for further human research.

Intermittent Fasting Can Increase Your Lifespan, Letting You Live longer

Some of the intermittent fasting's most promising uses may be its potential to prolong lifespan. Studies in rats have also shown that IF increases lifespan in a similar manner to constant restriction of calories. These variations in hormones, gene expression & cell function are linked to many of the advantages of intermittent fasting.

CHAPTER 3:

Reduce Hunger Pain During IF

You can expect to experience some feelings of hunger while you get used to your new eating schedule. Hunger has far less to do with the amount of food in your stomach than you might think. It is largely a function of your blood sugar levels, not how much or when you last ate. When your blood sugar is high, your body releases specific hormones that signal your brain to stop eating; they send the message that you are full. When your blood sugar drops, your body will release different hormones. The easiest way to successfully fast without experiencing too much hunger is to try to keep your blood sugar levels from fluctuating too drastically each day.

Ghrelin is the hormone that is responsible for making you feel hungry. These hormones are the kind that signal to your body that you are hungry and need food. It releases gastric acid into the stomach and causes hunger. This hormone usually peaks at its highest level around breakfast, lunch, and dinnertime. When you first start fasting, your ghrelin levels will continue to peak, and you will likely feel hungry. During fasting periods, try to avoid seeing or smelling food to prevent triggering this release.

There is a noticeable difference between physical hunger and emotional hunger. If you pay close attention to your body, you can start to recognize the subtle differences. Knowing the difference between physical and psychological hunger can assist with weight loss. It can lead you to make better choices, such as eating for the right reasons.

Physical hunger usually comes gradually and can be postponed for some amount of time. When you are physically hungry, you can satisfy it by eating any type of food. Once you are full, you generally feel satisfied, and you stop eating. Emotional hunger, on the other hand, may come on suddenly and feel more intense. It may lead to specific cravings, often for foods that are not good for you. When you are eating for emotional reasons, you may eat more than you normally would, and end up feeling uncomfortably full. Emotional eating often leaves you feeling guilty or bad about yourself.

You may find that you are not hungry one minute, but then are triggered by something in your environment and find yourself intensely hungry the next. Hunger itself is a conditioned response; it is something that you learn. You get hungry for many reasons such as smelling something good or going to an event that you have clearly associated with food. We are conditioned by many things in our environment to think about food constantly. Advertising especially reminds us of food constantly throughout the day. The good news is that the association that you have made between food and specific places and events in your life can be broken.

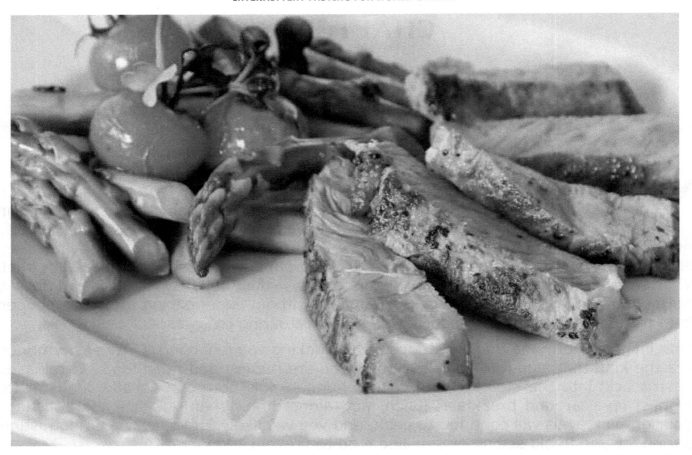

Eating a set number of meals each day is also a learned behavior; history tells us that it is not actually required. If you consistently eat at the same time every day, then the time of day itself will also be something that triggers your hunger. You condition yourself to become hungry at certain times of the day because of your own habits. Fasting will help you break yourself from the habit of eating three big meals a day. By skipping some meals and varying the times and the intervals at which you eat, you can program your body to eat when you are hungry, not because of the clock.

Dealing with hunger pain can become a challenge of mind over matter. Often, when you think you are hungry, it is just in your head. One strategy that can be very helpful is to try to maintain a positive mindset. When you feel the first pangs of hunger, try not to focus too much on it, or to start thinking about when you will have your next meal.

There are several additional strategies that you can use to help deal with your hunger when fasting.

- During non-fasting days, make sure to eat a balanced diet that contains a variety of proteins, fats, and carbohydrates.
- Make sure you consume your full days' worth of calories during eating windows; this will keep hunger at bay during fasting periods.
- Learn to tell the difference between hunger and thirst.
- Drink coffee and herbal tea to help alleviate hunger.
- Drink plenty of water; add flavor to your water as a treat.
- Chew sugarless gum if you feel like a snack.
- Brush your teeth; this is known to offset hunger pains.

- Stay active, busy, productive, and distracted.
- Get a healthy amount of sleep.

People who intermittently fast are often surprised that they are not as hungry as they think they will be when they change their eating patterns. This lifestyle plan is often easier than people think because it requires you to cut back on your food intake only for a limited amount of time. The rest of the time, you can eat normally and not feel hungry. Hunger pains when fasting are often less likely than they are with other diets. This could be because fasting allows blood sugar levels to stay more balanced. The hunger pains that are associated with most diets are what cause people to binge eat while trying to cut out calories.

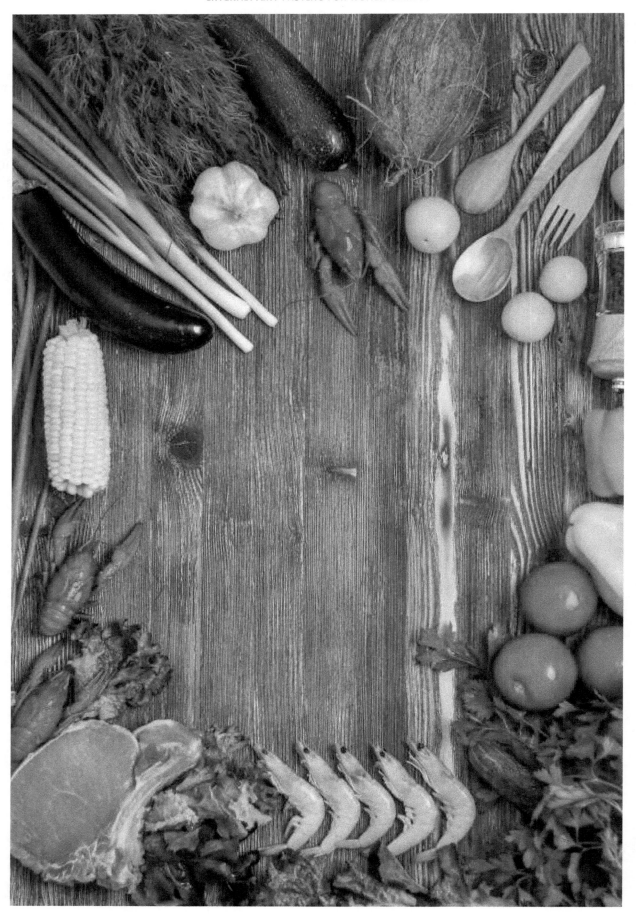

CHAPTER 4:

IF—Best Tips and Tricks

If you have gotten past the age of 50, you may begin to have health concerns and would want to maintain a body weight that is healthy as well as maximize the quality of your life. Just as is with everything else, there is no such thing as being "too old" to begin to live on a better diet, have better health, and fitness. The phrase, "Losing weight after 50" might sound like a lot of work, but the good news is that as a person advances in age, they have more wisdom and discipline, and if they put it to work, they can successfully lose a couple of pounds even past the age of 50.

Healthy Habits for Women Over 50

Loss of weight when you are past the age of 50 goes beyond engaging in regular exercise and following any kind of diet. There are other habits that, when developed, can play a significant role in improving your health and wellness, and particularly your mental health. The following are the healthy habits to develop:

Prioritize Brain Health

When people get older than 50 years, they begin to forget things easily and there is a decline in their cognitive abilities, which is normal for people at that age; and for women, this can be a very big concern. As a result, experts recommend that women over the age of 50 should exercise their brains just like they should do to every other muscle in their bodies. Do the following:

- Read regularly.
- Do crossword puzzles.
- Do more thinking about your career and try to comprehend a lot about it.
- Do tasks that involve math, such as balancing checkbooks and doing taxes.

When you ensure that your brain and thinking abilities remain sharp, you will improve your health and wellness in general.

Take Dietary Supplements

When you consume dietary supplements, it will help improve the functionality of your brain, enhance your mental health, reduce the risk of chronic diseases, especially osteoporosis and heart diseases, and avoid nutrient deficiencies. Below are a few supplements to consider:

- 500 milligrams of DHA plus EPA. This will help enhance cognitive function and boost heart health.
- 1-10 billion colony forming units (CFUs) of probiotics. This boosts immune function, improves the health of the skin, heart, and digestive system as well as eases anxiety and depression.

- 200 milligrams of green coffee bean extract, 3000 milligrams of Phaseolus Vulgaris (white kidney bean extract), or fiber supplements. They enhance weight loss, although you must discuss with your doctor and get their permission before consuming.
- Calcium, Vitamin D, and phosphorus supplements boost your bone health.
- 425 milligrams of choline. This improves brain function.
- Multivitamin supplements contain all essential vitamins and minerals including 150 micrograms of iodine made for women over the age of 50.

Before you take any dietary supplements, first check with your physician.

Get Enough Sleep

Getting enough sleep is important for persons of all ages. However, for older women, it is critically important. Women who have gone beyond the age of 50 should sleep for about 7 to 9 hours every night as recommended by the Centres for Disease Control and Prevention (CDC).

Sleep helps to check the hormones in the body that control appetite; it also prevents injury, boosts cognitive function, and energizes you for the activity of the day.

Focus on Mental Health

Besides taking supplements, healthy eating, exercise, and sleep, there are other things that you could do to reduce stress and anxiety. They include:

- Yoga.
- Meditation.
- Tai Chi.
- Outdoor walks and hikes.
- Getting a massage.
- Social support or talk therapy for depression.
- Get in touch with your spirituality.

Consult your physician when you can't get rid of anxiety, stress, or depression and see if they can recommend any medication for you.

Have Your Hormones Checked

Hormone levels tend to fluctuate when women age, especially during or after menopause. Therefore, when you hit 30, have your doctor monitor the following hormones:

- Estrogen.
- Progesterone.
- Thyroid hormone.

Abnormally low or high hormones can affect the metabolism of the body as well as the ability to lose weight. Consult your doctor and see if you should take isoflavone supplements or participate in hormone replacement therapy. Research shows that at least 75mgs of soy-derived isoflavones increase bone mineral density, enhances heart health, and could alleviate hot flushes that accompany menopause.

Drink Water, Coffee, and Tea

To prevent the fatigue that accompanies dehydration, as well as reduce hunger, drink a lot of water (about 2 to 4 cups) every morning after you wake up. Also, drink 2 cups of water before eating—it enhances satiation.

According to research, caffeine helps with weight loss. It further enhances mental alertness and boosts energy for exercise or daily activity. Drink 3 cups or more of coffee or tea every day (it is safe for most adults to drink 500 milligrams of caffeine a day).

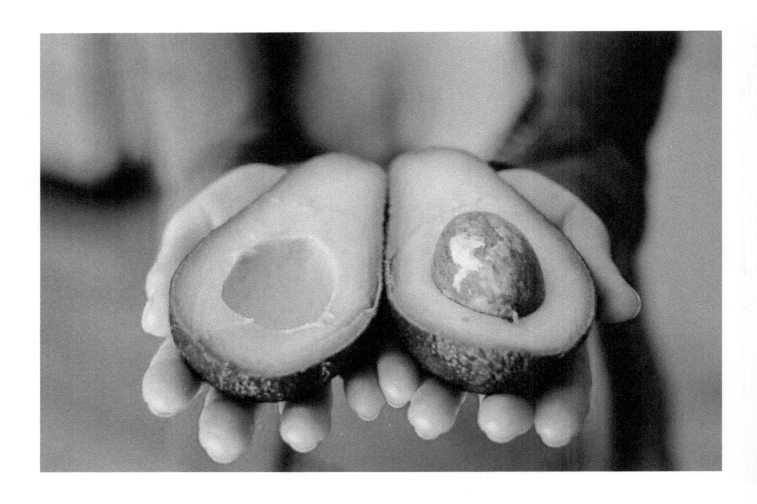

CHAPTER 5:

Most Mistakes to Avoid During IF

Don't Be Greedy in Festive Windows

The food has its temptation. It seems the most attractive thing in the world when it has been private for a long time. This would also happen to you. But it is important not to be greedy in those moments and lose control. It is very important to leave the windows fasting properly. The biggest mistake people make is that they eat a lot after breaking the fast. This can cause several problems, and poor digestion is one of them.

Do Not Try to Speed Up the Process

Slow and steady wins the race. This is an adage that we have all heard, but most of us do not believe. We want fast results, and for this, we are ready to jump. However, this is not how the body works. Your body travels very slowly. You need time to adapt to any positive or negative change, and the same would happen even in the case of intermittent fasting. If you want to succeed with the process, you must make sure you complete all the steps. You have to give your body time to adapt.

Perseverance Is the Key

Impatience is a big problem in people struggling with weight. There is no fault of them since they are subject to strong pressure. Most people trying to lose weight have already faced disappointments with other weight loss measures and want to see the results quickly to believe it. They are not ready to wait long for the results. This is a point where problems can occur. Intermittent fasting is not an excellent process. It is a wonderful process, but it does not work by magic. Try to correct problems that may have reached their current state of development in at least decades. The results would take time to arrive. You will have to work with patience and not lose hope when the results arrive. If you stop smoking in the middle, you cannot know if you are progressing or not. It is not a process that works overnight. A leap of faith will be required, and you will devote your time and energy.

Don't Frame Unrealistic Expectations

We all like to dream big, and that is a good thing. However, we must also remain based on reality. This will help to accept the facts and save many disappointments. Many times, we are so caught up in imaginary expectations that we don't recognize the gifts we receive. If your goal is weight loss, think about the amount of time you are ready to devote, the distances you can travel, and the medical conditions you face. Without considering all these facts, expecting a complete makeover would be absurd. If you have met these expectations, you will not even enjoy the weight loss you are observing. Your expectations would overshadow the results. It is important to stay realistic.

Properly Manage Your Fasting Time

It is not unusual for some people to mishandle their time. Many of us do it in our daily lives. However, bad time management can cause serious difficulties. It can make your weight loss journey difficult and painful. You can't keep thinking about food while you fast. This would create problems for you, and your gut would also be confused. The best way to manage your fasting time is to keep busy. The last part of the fasting window should always be programmed to remain locked correctly. The more inactive it is, the more likely it is to think only of food. Performing intense physical activity is one of the best ways to postpone hunger.

CHAPTER 6:

The Fasting and Hormone Connection

As you know by now, when you fast, your body adjusts itself to make its fat stores more accessible for use. This is a response to the starvation that the cells experience, but this can happen without the human experiencing starvation. It does this by adjusting hormone levels. The human body reacts as if it were experiencing starvation at a cellular level to anticipate a possible absence of food. This environment that intermittent fasting creates in the body leads to a release of hormones that have beneficial effects on the body.

Insulin

Intermittent fasting leads to lower levels of insulin active in the bloodstream during fasting periods (due to less food, specifically sugars being taken into the body) that then leads to improved use of fat cells for energy which, over time, increases the effectiveness of insulin, which is one of the main hormones involved in metabolism, as it signals to cells that there has been an intake in sugar and awakens them to process and store this sugar. By reducing the sugar, the insulin becomes more sensitive to the environment of the body, and over time, this is beneficial for the insulin cells and blood sugar levels of the woman practicing intermittent fasting.

Further, when insulin levels are lower, this leads to the release of another hormone called HGH, which also helps in the breakdown and use of stored fat cells for energy, which leads to weight loss.

Another hormone that is triggered by intermittent fasting is Norepinephrine or Noradrenaline, which becomes released in response to an empty stomach. This hormone encourages the release and the metabolism of fat cells for energy, which also leads to weight loss and improved health due to a reduction in belly fat often found in women over 50.

The Menstrual Cycle

When fasting, some women have experienced changes in their menstrual cycle. The bodies of women are more sensitive to small-calorie changes, especially when it comes to a reduction in calorie intake. Since the bodies of women are built to conceive and grow babies, their bodies have to be sensitive to changes in the internal environment to a larger degree than the bodies of men. When the bodies of women experience a reduction in calorie intake, they may have trouble experiencing regular menstrual cycles as the body may deem the internal environment less than ideal for a baby to be grown. This is not to say that women cannot practice Intermittent Fasting or fasting of any sort, but that they must keep this in mind when deciding to try a fasting diet.

Intermittent Fasting and Menopause

Intermittent fasting in women has been shown to lead to the release of hormones that, in turn, lead to the release of bone minerals such as phosphate and calcium, and the release of these bone minerals leads to increase bone density and strength, which is especially beneficial in women who are over 50, as the risk of developing osteoporosis is very high. Therefore, inducing autophagy in the body leads to a reduction in the risk of developing osteoporosis in women over 50, and can even lead to improvements in women who have already been diagnosed with it.

When it comes to menopause, many things in your body can feel like they are out of your control. Menopause can lead to weight gain, depression, anxiety, increased risk of heart disease, among others. It will also lead to changes in the hormones and the metabolism of the women that are in menopause, as well as a reduction in the body's sensitivity to insulin.

Because of all of these side effects that come with menopause, intermittent fasting has been tested as a method for reducing those side effects and has shown to be useful in improving them. Intermittent fasting has proven to be a good choice for improving the symptoms of menopause, such as the pesky weight gain that many women experience, reducing the risk of heart disease and depression, as well as improved cognitive functioning. Therefore, not only can Intermittent Fasting improve the way you feel about your body and yourself in general during this time of transition, but it can also make you live a longer and healthier life.

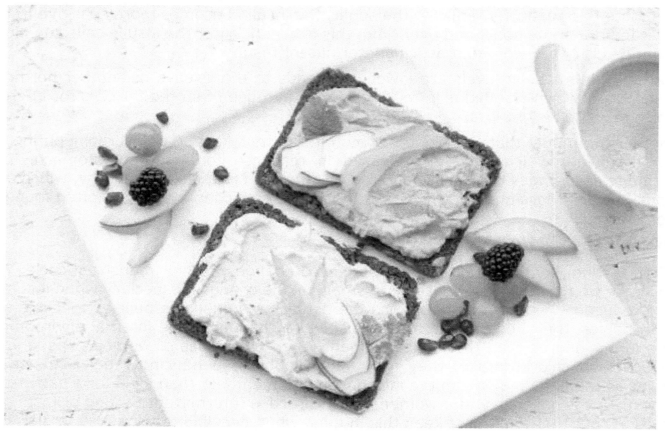

CHAPTER 7:

Diet in Menopause

Menopause is one of the most complicated phases in a woman's life. The time when our bodies begin to change and important natural transitions occur that are too often negatively affected, while it is important to learn how to change our eating habits and eating patterns appropriately. In fact, it often happens that a woman is not ready for this new condition and experiences it with a feeling of defeat as an inevitable sign of time travel, and this feeling of prostration turns out to be too invasive and involves many aspects of one's stomach. It is, therefore, important to remain calm as soon as there are messages about the first signs of change in our human body to ward off the onset of menopause for the right purpose and to minimize the negative effects of suffering, especially in the early days. Even during this difficult transition, targeted nutrition can be very beneficial.

What Happens to The Body of a Menopausal Woman?

It must be said that a balanced diet has been carried out in life and there are no major weight fluctuations, this will no doubt be a factor that supports women who are going through menopause, but that it is not a sufficient condition to present with classic symptoms that are felt, which can be classified according to the period experienced. In fact, we can distinguish between the pre-menopausal phase, which lasts around 45 to 50 years, and is physiologically compatible with a drastic reduction in the production of the hormone estrogen (responsible for the menstrual cycle, which actually starts irregularly.) This period is accompanied by a series of complex and highly subjective endocrine changes. Compare effectively: headache, depression, anxiety, and sleep disorders.

When someone enters actual menopause, estrogen hormone production decreases even more dramatically and the range of the symptoms widens, leading to large amounts of the hormone, for example, to a certain class called catecholamine adrenaline. The result of these changes is a dangerous heat wave, increased sweating, and the presence of tachycardia, which can be more or less severe.

However, the changes also affect the female genital organs, with the volume of the breasts, uterus, and ovaries decreasing. The mucous membranes become less active and vaginal dryness increases. There may also be changes in bone balance, with decreased calcium intake and increased mobilization at the expense of the skeletal system. Because of this, there is a lack of continuous bone formation, and conversely, erosion begins, which is a predisposition for osteoporosis.

Although menopause causes major changes that greatly change a woman's body and soul, metabolism is one of the worst. In fact, during menopause, the absorption and accumulation of sugars and triglycerides change and it is easy to increase some clinical values such as cholesterol and triglycerides, which lead to high blood pressure or arteriosclerosis. In addition, many women often complain of disturbing circulatory disorders and local edema, especially in the stomach. It also makes weight gain easier, even though you haven't changed your eating habits.

The Ideal Diet for Menopause

In cases where disorders related to the arrival of menopause become difficult to manage, drug or natural therapy under medical supervision may be necessary. The contribution given by a correct diet at this time can be considerable;, given the profound variables that come into play, it is necessary to modify our food routine, both in order not to be surprised by all these changes and to adapt in the most natural way possible.

The problem of fat accumulation in the abdominal area is always caused by the drop in estrogen. In fact, they are also responsible for the classic hourglass shape of most women, which consists of depositing fat mainly on the hips, which begins to fail with menopause. As a result, we go from a gynoid condition to an android one, with an adipose increase localized on the belly. In addition, the metabolic rate of disposal is reduced, this means that even if you do not change your diet and eat the same quantities of food as you always have, you could experience weight gain, which will be more marked in the presence of bad habits or irregular diet. The digestion is also slower and intestinal function becomes more complicated. This further contributes to swelling as well as the occurrence of intolerance and digestive disorders that have never been disturbed before. Therefore, the beginning will be more problematic and difficult to manage during this period. The distribution of nutrients must be different: reducing the amount of low carbohydrate, which is always preferred not to be purified, helps avoid the peak of insulin and at the same time maintains stable blood sugar.

Furthermore, it will be necessary to slightly increase the quantity of both animal and vegetable proteins; choose good fats, preferring seeds and extra virgin olive oil, and severely limit saturated fatty acids (those of animal origin such as lard, lard, etc.). All this to try to increase the proportion of antioxidants taken, which will help to counteract the effect of free radicals which concentration begins to increase during this period. It will be necessary to prefer foods rich in phytoestrogens, which will help to control the states of stress to which the body is subjected, and which will favor, at least in part, the overall estrogenic balance.

These molecules are divided into three main groups and the foods that contain them should never be missing on our tables: isoflavones, present mainly in legumes such as soy and red clover; lignans, of which flax seeds and oily seeds, in general, are particularly rich; cumestani, found in sunflower seeds, beans, and sprouts. A calcium supplementation will be necessary through cheeses such as parmesan; dairy products such as yogurt, egg yolk, some vegetables such as rocket, Brussels sprouts, broccoli, spinach, asparagus; legumes; dried fruit such as nuts, almonds, or dried grapes.

Excellent additional habits that will help to regain well-being may be limiting sweets to sporadic occasions, thus drastically reducing sugars (for example, by giving up sugar in coffee and getting used to drinking it bitterly); learn how to dose alcohol a lot (avoiding spirits, liqueurs, and aperitif drinks) and choose only one glass of good wine when you are in company. This because it tends to increase visceral fat, which is precisely what is going to settle at the level abdominal. Clearly, even by eating lots of fruit, it is difficult to reach a high carbohydrate quota as in a traditional diet. However, a dietary plan to follow can be useful to have a more precise indication of how to distribute the foods. Obviously, one's diet must be structured in a personal way, based on specific metabolic needs and one's lifestyle.

CHAPTER 8:

IF and Keto: Could You Combine the Two?

The idea behind intermittent fasting is to provide your body with an extended fasting period, allowing it to enter into a state of ketosis. Intermittent fasting is a lifestyle and dieting method that has gained popularity in the past few years for its effectiveness in weight loss. However, many people are unclear on how best to implement intermittent fasting concerning the ketogenic diet (keto). In this article, we'll review some of the most common questions people have when combining these two methods and give you our take on how they could be combined.

Why Would You Want to Do This?

Advantages of Intermittent Fasting

The usual reason people decide to go on "intermittent fasts" is because they want to lose weight. Perhaps they follow a low-carb diet and find that if they don't break their fast periodically, the effects of ketosis are not lasting enough. Or perhaps they want to increase their caloric intake to prepare for training. Oftentimes, people will break fasting periods by having a high-carb meal or refueling with a protein shake. However, one of the most significant benefits of intermittent fasting is weight loss.

Intermittent Fasting and Dieting

Experienced intermittent fasters can lose up to 13 pounds in 12 weeks without reducing calories or doing any exercise. That's an average of over 1 pound lost per week—and that's without any workout program at all. With normal calorie consumption, this could result in significant weight loss for a year.

Intermittent Fasting and Exercise

Many intermittent faster find that their bodies become leaner while they exercise, even at the same calorie intake. This is because the body fat percentage decreases while muscle mass increases. Also, many people who are new to dieting may find that intermittent fasting makes it easier to deal with hunger pangs.

Intermittent Fasting and Keto Dieting

While intermittent fasting can be a great way to lose weight, it's not necessarily good for ketosis. If the body is in a state of ketosis and you fast for a while, you could risk breaking this state.

Intermittent Fasting and Workout Performance

Many people report that intermittent fasting has a positive effect on their workouts. In one study of boxers, it was discovered that using alternate-day fasting (alternating 24-hour fasting with eating days) allowed them to train harder on their exercise days because they maintained more muscle glycogen than the control group did (who ate 3 meals per day).

The Issue of Muscle Loss

The belief that intermittent fasting causes the body to break down muscle mass is a myth. It is true that when you fast, your blood sugar could drop to levels that would make you feel tired and hungry. However, this would only be the case if your body was not in ketosis. The reason behind this is because insulin levels do not rise significantly during intermittent fasting, even with large amounts of carbohydrates in the diet. Once in ketosis, insulin levels will be so low that it's not possible for blood sugar levels to feel too low to cause hunger or fatigue (unless you are going for long periods without eating anything at all). This is because the body will be using ketone bodies for energy, not sugar.

Intermittent Fasting and Hunger

If you're a chronic calorie-counter or someone who is not good at controlling their eating, you may feel hungrier during intermittent fasts. When people try to do low or no-carb diets in the past, they often blame keto side effects on carb cravings. Whether or not you are actually being affected by carb cravings during ketosis, depends on factors such as your dietary choices before initiating a ketogenic diet and your ability to control food intake.

Intermittent Fasting and Thirst

There is some evidence that intermittent fasting could increase your risk for dehydration. Both of the studies reviewed by a 2017 study found that there was a link between both insufficient intake of water and increased urinary ketone bodies. However, it's not known whether this increase in urine ketones is due to an increase in the body trying to excrete ketones or an increase in water loss through the urine.

Intermittent Fasting and Fatigue

Some people claim that intermittent fasting makes them feel fatigued or worn out during the day. This would be especially true if you're eating a very low-carb diet (3% or less) without any calories. If you're following a high-carb diet with intermittent fasting, you're likely consuming far fewer calories, which means the body uses more fat and glycogen as fuel.

Intermittent Fasting and Insulin Secretion

It has been suggested that having too little glucose in the blood could reduce insulin secretion. This could potentially decrease the effectiveness of the ketogenic diet. If you are someone who tends to be highly sensitive to insulin, this could be a problem for you (see this post for more information).

Intermittent Fasting and Omega-3

Some people who follow a ketogenic diet notice that they don't feel as good as they should. There is some evidence that the omega-3 fatty acids in animal foods are linked to better brain function and can help with depression. This could be because many people aren't getting enough omega-3 fatty acids in their diets. Eating eggs, sardines, anchovies, or taking cod liver oil while on a ketogenic diet could help with this problem.

CHAPTER 9:

Types of IF

16:8 Method

The 16:8 method is one of the most popular methods among Intermittent Fasters. Essentially, you spend 16 hours within each day fasting, and the other 8 hours are your eating window. Most people try to choose their 8-hour eating window to be the times when they're primarily active. If you're a night person, feel free to make it a little later.

Hold off eating during the daytime as much as possible and then breakfast around 3 or 4 pm. For morning people, breakfast earlier, say, around 11 am, stopping food consumption by 7 pm.

This method is incredibly flexible and works for many different kinds of people. It's even flexible once you decide to try a particular fasting to the eating window ratio. For example, if you don't seem to be jiving with the 11–7 pm eating window, you can absolutely alter the next day to suit your needs better. Maybe try waiting until later in the day for breakfast! Try what you need to do as long as you're keeping to that 16:8-hour ratio.

Whereas the lean-gains method technically applies the same hourly ratio, it's much stricter regarding a healthy diet and exercise regimen. The 16:8 method does not need any type of exercise booster, but that's up to the practitioner. It is always best to try adding healthy dietary choices to one's IF eating schedule but don't try to restrict too many calories, as it can incorporate feelings of lightheadedness and low energy. With 16:8, you can eat what you need and swap the hours around as desired.

The Warrior Method

The warrior method is quite similar to the 20:4 method in that the individual fasts for 20 hours within each day and breaks fast for a 4-hour eating window. The difference is in the outlook and mindset of the practitioner, however. Essentially, the thought process behind the warrior method is that, in ancient times, the hunter coming home from stalking prey or the warrior coming home from battle would really only get one meal each day. One meal would have to provide sustenance for the rest of the day, recuperative energy from the ordeal, and sustainable energy for the future.

Therefore, practitioners of the warrior method are encouraged to have one large meal when they breakfast, and that meal should be jam-packed with fats, proteins, and carbs for the rest of the day (and for the days ahead). Just like with the 20:4 method, however, it can sometimes be too intense for practitioners, and it's very easy to scale this one back in forcefulness by making up a method like 18:6 or 17:7. If it's not working, don't force it to work past two weeks, but do try to make it through a week to see if it's your stubbornness or if it's just a mismatch with the method.

5:2 Method

5:2 method is popular among those who want to take things up a notch generally. Instead of fasting and eating within each day, these individuals take up a practice of fasting two whole days out of the week. The other 5 days are free to eat, exercise, or diet as desired, but those other two days (that can be consecutive or scattered throughout the week) must be strictly fasting days.

For those fasting days, it's not as if the individual can't eat anything altogether, however. In actuality, one is allowed to consume no more than 500 calories each day for this Intermittent Fasting method. I suppose these fasting days would be better referred to as "restricted-intake" days, for that is a more accurate description.

5:2 method is extremely rewarding, but it is also one of the more difficult ones to attempt. If you're having issues with this method, don't be afraid to experiment the next week with a method like 14:10 or 16:8, where you're fasting and eating within each day. If that works better for you, don't be ashamed to embrace it! However, if you're dedicated to having days "on" and days "off" with fasting and eating, there are other alternatives, too.

Eat-Stop-Eat (24-Hour) Method

The eat-stop-eat or 24-hour method is another option for people who want to have days "on" and "off" between fasting and eating. It's a little less intense than the 5:2 method, and it's much more flexible for the individual, based on what they need. For instance, if you need a literal 24-hour fast each week and that's it; you can do that. On the other hand, if you want a more flexible 5:2 method-type thing to happen, you can work with what you want and create a method surrounding those desires and goals.

The most successful approaches to the eat-stop-eat method have involved more strict dieting (or at the very least, cautious and healthy eating) during the 5 or 6 days when the individual engages in the week's free-eating window. For the individual to truly see success with weight loss, there will have to be some caloric restriction (or high nutrition focus) those 5 or 6 days, too, so that the body will have a version of consistency in health and nutrition content.

On the one or two days each week that the individual decides to fast, there can still be highly restricted caloric intake. As with the 5:2 method, they can consume no more than 500 calories worth of food and drink during these fasting days so that the body can maintain energy flow and more.

If the individual engages in exercise, those workout days should absolutely be reserved for the 5 or 6 free-eating days. The same goes for the 5:2 method. Try not to exercise (at least not excessively) on those days that are chosen for fasting. Your body will not appreciate the added stress when you're taking in so few calories. As always, you can choose to move up from eat-stop-eat to another method if this works easily and you're interested in something more. Furthermore, you can start with a strict 24-hour method and then move up to a more flexible eat-stop-eat approach! Do what feels right, and never be afraid to troubleshoot one method for the sake of choosing another.

Alternate-Day Method

The alternate-day method is similar to the eat-stop-eat and 5:2 methods because it focuses on individual days "on" and "off" for fasting and eating. The difference for this method, in particular, is that it ends up being at least 2 days a week fasting, and sometimes, it can be as many as 4.

Some people follow very strict approaches to the alternate-day method and literally fast every other day, only consuming 500 calories or less on those days designated for fasting. Some people, on the other hand, are much more flexible, and they tend to go for two days eating, one day fasting, two days eating, one day fasting, etc. The alternate-day method is even more flexible than eat-stop-eat in that sense for it allows the individual to choose how they alternate between eating and fasting, based on what works for the body and mind the best.

The alternate-day method is like a step up from eat-stop-eat and 24-hour methods, especially if the individual truly alternates one-day fasting and the next day eating, etc. This more intense style of fasting works particularly well for people who are working on equally intense fitness regimens, surprisingly. People who are eating more calories a day than 2000 (which is true for a lot of bodybuilders and fitness buffs) will have more to gain from the alternate-day method, for you only have to cut back your eating on fasting days to about 25 percent of your standard caloric intake. Therefore, those fasting days can still provide solid nutritional support for fitness experts while helping them sculpt their bodies and maintain a new level of health.

Spontaneous Skipping Method

The alternate-day method and eat-stop-eat method are certainly flexible in their approaches to when the individual fasts and when they eat. However, none of those mentioned above plans are quite as flexible as the spontaneous skipping method. The spontaneous skipping method literally only requires that the individual skip meals within each day, whenever desired—and when it's sensed that the body can handle it.

Many people with more sensitive digestive systems or who practice more intense fitness regimens will start their experiences with IF through the spontaneous skipping method before moving on to something more intensive. People who have very haphazard daily schedules or who are around food a lot but forget to eat will benefit from this method, for it works well with chaotic schedules and unplanned energies.

Despite that chaotic and unorganized potential, the spontaneous skipping method can also be more structured and organized, depending on what you make of it! For instance, someone desiring more structure can choose what meal each day they'd like to skip. Let's say they choose to skip breakfast each day. Then, their spontaneous skipping method will be structured around making sure to skip breakfast (a.k.a.—not to eat until at least 12 pm) daily. Whatever you need to do to make this method work, try it! This method is made for experimentation and adventurousness.

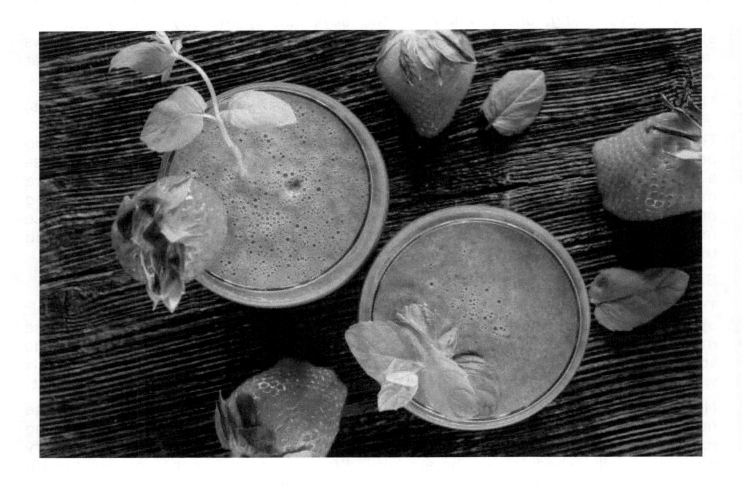

CHAPTER 10:

Exercise to Support IF

Exercises to Do With Intermittent Fasting in Women Over 50

Two forms of exercise, aerobic and anaerobic, are essential. Exercise for a prolonged time, such as racing, biking, and swimming, is physical exercise, or "cardio" anaerobic training, such as weight lifting or sprinting, involves full intensity for a limited time.

The type of exercise an individual performs is likely to depend on the type of intermittent fasting they practice. For instance, an individual doing nightly fasts or 16:8 will do either anaerobic exercise or aerobic exercise during their eating while not over-exerting themselves. If anyone does alternate days and wishes to work out on their day of fasting, they should usually adhere to physical exercise less severe. Two main things to look out for if you want to try an exercise with intermittent fasting:

- **Timing of the workout:** while an individual can work out in a fasting state, it may be easier to exercise after meals.
- **Sort of food:** it is necessary to know what to consume while exercising throughout times of consumption.

The nutrition of pre-workout consists of consuming a meal 2–3 hours before doing exercise rather than just before exercising. It should be high in complex carbs, such as protein and cereal from whole grains. A post-workout meal should consist of fresh vegetables, good-quality proteins, and fats to facilitate healing. For some people over 50, fasting and exercising daily might be dangerous, including:

- People who had disordered eating.
- People with low blood pressure.
- People with heart condition.
- People with diabetes.

If an individual has just worked out: the meal they consume should be 50 to 60 percent of the calories in this situation and have a mixture of macronutrients.

If an individual is working out later: the meal they consume should be 30 to 50 percent of the calories in the meal, made up of a combination of macronutrients.

When an individual has existing health problems but needs to try the intermittent fasting and work out, it is better to speak to the doctor.

Light Movement Exercise During Intermittent Fasting Include

- Rather than laying or sitting still, light movement is good.
- Get up and making a cup of coffee and tea.
- Moving around the building.

- Strolling at a steady speed.
- Dusting and washing.
- Vacuuming activities.
- Make your bed.
- Walking and standing than walking.
- Yoga.

Examples of Moderately Intense Activities

- Water aerobics.
- Riding a bicycle.
- Walking briskly.
- Dancing like exercise.
- Hiking on a hill.
- Playing doubles tennis.
- Push a lawnmower.

These are some excises that women over 50 can also try with intermittent fasting:

- **Aerobic exercises:** includes running, jogging, walking, cycling, and dance activity are good things to do. Aerobic activity works with the body's broad muscles, aiding the cardiovascular system, and losing weight. Work up to having 20 minutes or more, a session, and 3 to 4 days each week. Be sure you can pass the "talk test," which involves exercising at a speed that lets you continue on a conversation.
- **Strength exercises:** lifting hand weights strengthens stamina and balance, improves bone strength, decreases the likelihood of lower back injuries, and makes you fit. Begin with a hand weight that you can easily handle for eight repetitions. Add more reps progressively before you can total 12.
- **Stretching:** stretching movements aim to preserve joint stability and range of motion. They often reduce the likelihood of muscle soreness and injuries. Pilates and yoga is a good way of stretching exercise, strengthening the core body, and enhancing flexibility.

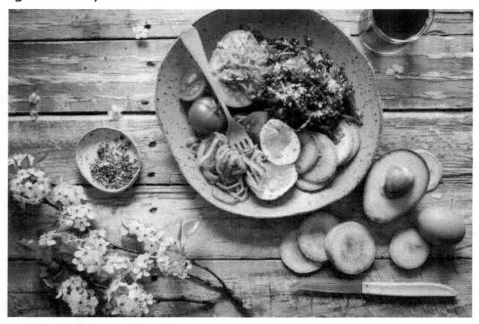

CHAPTER 11:

Meditation and IF Combined

This should come as no surprise that most women who pick up a method to lose weight surrender midway. Make no mistake, losing weight is a daunting task, and the body is not ready to give up the fat it loves so dearly. This means that you can witness periods of no progress. When people are faced with such patches, they lose all their conviction and motivation. They completely stop making an effort and return to their old ways. The result is not hard to guess. You must understand that losing weight can be hard. You may face several challenges on the way, and there may come several phases when you would want to throw the towel. However, that's the time you need motivation and support.

Finding motivation is very important for the success of any weight loss effort. We all are human beings, and there would be times when you would feel low and would want to give up. In those times, if there is someone to counsel and provide support, your weight loss journey would get easier. Usually, this is the toughest thing to do for people trying to lose weight. They fear getting laughed at, ridiculed, or judged. This is a situation that you will have to be prepared for.

Confide in Someone

You must have someone with whom you can discuss your progress and talk about your efforts. You can confide in a close friend, family member, or anyone else you think would be supportive and understanding. It is not the counseling that one needs in depressing situations but a shoulder to lean on.

Ensure You Are in a Conducive Environment

This is another important thing that you need to look for. Fasting can be tough at times, and if you are on any specific diet surrounded by people who are eating all the time and specifically eating the things you can't or won't want to eat can be difficult. An easy way out of this problem is to inform your family members about your efforts so that you don't have to face eating people while you are in the fasting period. This lowers the chances of temptation.

Support Groups

Support groups can also be helpful in such efforts. You can join a support group and find other people struggling with similar issues. Such groups can be very helpful in sharing problems and understanding the common impediments that can come in the way. Support groups help you understand the issues others have faced and that can also ease the pain you may be feeling. Most of the time, when we are dealing with a problem and there are no other experiences in front of us as a reference point, our problems start looking very big. The sharing of problems in the support groups helps in building a wider and better perspective.

Seek Professional Help

This is another medium you can use. Several clinics can help you dealing with the problem, and they can also provide expert guidance in case you are also dealing with other underlying issues. You can consult clinics that can help in tracking your progress so that staying motivated can become more objective.

Meditation and Positive Affirmations

Meditation is a great way to stay motivated. It is a healthy way to build positive energy inside you and chase away the negative thoughts. Practicing meditation for a few minutes daily can help you in staying motivated. You can also use positive affirmations to keep yourself motivated. There is scientific evidence behind the fact that repeating positive things can help driving away from the stress from the mind, and it makes us feel good. Therefore, if you tend to feel demotivated quickly, taking the help of positive affirmations can be very helpful.

CHAPTER 12:

Shopping List

Meal prep might seem a bit challenging at first, but just remember you don't need to prep all of your meals at one time. You can begin with the meats one evening and veggies the next; it's all up to you! The segment using veggies in this book is prepared to use within a couple of days (unless otherwise shown).

Decide How to Prep

Do you want to prepare all of the chicken, pork, or other meal selections one night and the veggies the next night? Or do you want to cook each meal individually but in bulk? No worries, either way, each of the recipes has instructions for individual prep tips as well. Purchase the containers you want to use. These are some guidelines for those:

- Mason Jars—pint or quart size.
- Ziploc—type freezer bags.
- Rubbermaid Stackable—Glad Containers.
- Microwavable.
- Freezer Safe.
- Stackable.
- BPA Free.
- Reusable.

Label the Containers

There are some other things you have to consider when freezing your meals. You should always label your container with the date that you put it in the freezer. You also need to double-check that your bottles, jars, or bags are each sealed tightly. If your containers aren't air-tight, your food will become freezer burnt and need to be trashed.

Set Aside Quiet Time for Prep Day

Choose a time when you won't have any interruptions.

Inventory the Kitchen

Buy your food in bulk to reduce the cost. Saving money while on the ketogenic diet is vital. Purchasing your items in bulk can make a severe impact. Check your area for local farms that raise their animals on pasture feeding or a local market for fresh produce. After you find a good deal, stock up and purchase pantry items such as seasonings and flour. You can freeze many things and save a bundle of cash.

Select Your Meal Plan

You will begin with your 30-day plan and build from there. As you proceed with your daily selections, make notes of which ones you enjoyed the most and the ones you want to omit for your next month's planning.

Chop Your Veggies in Advance

Prepare and freeze plenty of healthy fruits and yogurt into a delicious smoothie for the entire week. Enjoy one for breakfast or any time you have the craving. Purchase foods in bulk to be used for taco meats, breakfast burritos, fajita fillings, soups, egg muffins, and so much more. As you prep, include lean proteins for the weekends in a container for a quick grab 'n' go snack or luncheon for a weekend journey.

Tips for Vegetable & Meat Selections

Select Fresh Meats and Dairy When Possible

Try to find meat and dairy that has an expiration date for as far in the future as possible. These choices will tend to remain fresh and last longer. This also applies to the "sell by" dates. The further in the future, either of these dates is, the surer you can bet that the food is going to last the week.

Select Whole Not Chopped Meats & Veggies

You can save big by chopping your own meats and vegetables. You will pay for the person that is doing the cutting for your convenience.

Freeze & Reheat Your Meals

For meals that are scheduled to be eaten at least three days after cooking, freezing is a great option. Freezing food is safe and convenient, but it doesn't work for every type of meal. You can also freeze the ingredients for a slow cooker meal and then just dump out the container into the slow cooker and leave it there. This saves a lot of time and means you can pre-prep meals up to 1–2 months in advance.

The last food safety consideration you need to make with regards to meal prepping is how you reheat food. Most people opt to microwave their meals for warming, but you can use any other conventional heating source in your kitchen as well. The reason people love the microwave for heating their meal prep meals is that it's quick and convenient.

However, you have to be careful with microwaving because over-cooking can cause food to taste bad. To combat this, cook your food in one-minute intervals and check on it between each minute. You can also help your food cook more evenly and quickly but keeping your meat cut into small pieces when you cook it. You should never put frozen food directly from the freezer into the microwave. Let your frozen food thaw first.

Food reheating and prep safety will become second nature over time. Meal prep is challenging when you are just starting out but becomes much simpler after you have seen it done. Some errors can be avoided.

However, mistakes do happen, and as such, it's best to cook for short periods rather than longer ones, so you have less of a risk of making a mistake and needing to scrap everything you have prepared for that substantial time. While it is a lot and seems complicated, meal prepping is the best way to set yourself up for success with the keto diet.

Example of How Meal Prep Works

Choose Healthy Produce

Carrots, red bell peppers, cucumbers, baby spinach, and any other keto-friendly veggies you prefer.

Protein Options

Two cans of tuna, one pound of lunch meat of your choice (turkey, ham, roast beef), and two pounds of skinless chicken thighs or one pound of salmon (this will be used for lunch and dinner)

Dairy Options

Cheese sticks (of your choice), heavy cream, sour cream, grass-fed butter, keto-friendly salad dressing, mayo, mustard, and eggs.

Dry Goods Options

Coffee, avocado oil, pecans, almonds, salt, pepper, and your seasonings of choice.

Method of Preparation

From there, you will do the following steps to prepare your lunch and dinner for the week:

1. Get ten plastic containers ready to fill with your meals.
2. Chop up vegetables and put them in five different plastic containers.
3. Combine baby spinach salad with vegetables of choice to make five salads.
4. Boil eggs and peel.
5. Mix the canned tuna with mayo, mustard, salt, and pepper. Put the tuna salad in two different plastic containers that already have a salad or mixed vegetables in them.
6. Bake four pieces of chicken and four pieces of salmon. Season it with your seasonings of choice and cook them in avocado oil.
7. Combine four pieces of salmon and four pieces of chicken with the ten containers that are already filled with salad and chopped vegetables.
8. Finish the ten meals by adding your choice of pecans, almonds, hard-boiled eggs, and cheese sticks. These will be snacks to supplement your meals.

You are ready to go and prepare all of your breakfast, lunch, and dinner for the coming week. This method takes 2 to 3 hours and provides well-balanced meals for each of the seven nights of the week.

CHAPTER 13:

Top Foods to Eat and Drink IF Benefits, 14 Day Meal Plan

Breakfast

1. Healthy Chia and Oats Smoothie

Preparation Time: 10 minutes.

Cooking Time: 0 minutes

Servings: 2

Ingredients:

- 6 tbsps. oats.
- 2 tbsps. chia seeds.
- 2 tbsps. hemp powder.
- 4 Medjool dates, pitted (optional).
- 2 bananas, chopped.
- 1 cup almond milk.
- 1 cup frozen berries.
- 2 big handful's spinach, torn.

Directions:

1. Add all the ingredients to a blender and blend until smooth.
2. Pour in glasses and serve.

Nutrition:

- **Calories:** 140.
- **Fat:** 7 g.
- **Fiber:** 4 g.
- **Carbs:** 12 g.
- **Protein:** 12 g.

2. Cherry Almond and Cereal Smoothie

Preparation Time: 10 minutes.

Cooking Time: 0 minutes.

Servings: 2

Ingredients:

- 1 cup fresh cherries, pitted + extra to garnish.
- ¼ cup rolled oats.
- 1 tbsp. hemp seeds.
- 1 cup almond milk.

Directions:

1. Add all the ingredients to a blender and blend until smooth.
2. Pour into glasses and serve garnished with cherries.

Nutrition:

- **Calories:** 200.
- **Fat:** 8 g.
- **Fiber:** 4 g.
- **Carbs:** 8 g.
- **Protein:** 3 g.

3. Banana Orange Smoothie

Preparation Time: 10 minutes.

Cooking Time: 0 minutes.

Servings: 2

Ingredients:

- 2 cups fat-free milk.
- 1 cup nonfat Greek yogurt.
- 1 medium banana.
- 1 cup collard greens.
- 1 orange, peeled, deseeded, separated into segments.
- 6 strawberries, chopped.
- 2 tbsps. sesame seeds.

Directions:

1. Add all the ingredients to a blender and blend until smooth.
2. Pour in glasses and serve.

Nutrition:

- **Calories:** 183.
- **Fat:** 8 g.
- **Fiber:** 1 g.
- **Carbs:** 3 g.
- **Protein:** 9 g.

4. Crunchy Banana Yoghurt

Preparation Time: 10 minutes

Cooking Time: 0 minutes

Servings: 4

Ingredients:

- 3 cups fat-free natural Greek-style yogurt.
- 1 oz. mixed seeds or nuts of your choice like pumpkin seeds etc.
- 2 bananas, sliced.

Directions:

1. Take 4 bowls and add ¾ cup yogurt into each bowl.
2. Divide the banana slices among the bowl.
3. Sprinkle seeds on top and serve.

Nutrition:

- **Calories:** 323.
- **Fat:** 11 g.
- **Fiber:** 4 g.
- **Carbs:** 13 g.
- **Protein:** 17 g.

5. Grapefruit Yogurt Parfait

Preparation Time: 10 minutes.

Cooking Time: 5 minutes.

Servings: 4

Ingredients:

- ½ cup amaranth.
- 1 grapefruit, peeled, separated into segments, deseeded, chopped.
- 3 tbsps. toasted coconut.
- Stevia to taste (optional).
- 1 cup plain, nonfat yogurt.

Directions:

1. Place a pan over medium heat. Add amaranth and let it pop. It should take 3–5 minutes. Let it cool for a few minutes.
2. Add yogurt into a bowl. Add stevia and stir. Add 2 tbsps. yogurt into each of 4 glasses.
3. Place a layer of grapefruit in each glass. Add 1 tbsp. popped amaranth and sprinkle some coconut into the glasses.
4. Repeat steps 2–3 until all the ingredients are used up.

Nutrition:

- **Calories:** 103 g.
- **Fat:** 4 g.
- **Fiber:** 1 g.
- **Carbs:** 3 g.
- **Protein:** 22 g.

6. Creamy Mango and Banana Overnight Oats

Preparation Time: 10 minutes.

Cooking Time: 0 minutes.

Servings: 1

Ingredients:

For the smoothie:

- 1 ripe banana.
- ½ mango, peeled, cubed.
- ½ tbsp. ground flaxseed.
- 1 cup almond milk.

For the oats:

- $1/3$ cup oats.
- 1 small ripe banana, mashed.
- ½ cup almond milk.
- ½ tbsp. ground flaxseed.
- 2 tbsps. chia seeds.
- Stevia or erythritol to taste.

Directions:

1. Add all the smoothie ingredients into a blender and blend until smooth.
2. Pour into a tall glass.

To make the oats layer:

1. Add oats, almond milk, flaxseed, chia seeds, and stevia into a bowl. Stir well and add banana. Mix until well combined. Pour it over the smoothie in the glass.
2. Chill in the refrigerator overnight and serve.

Nutrition:

- **Calories:** 199 g.
- **Fat:** 8 g.
- **Fiber:** 4 g.
- **Carbs:** 9 g.
- **Protein:** 4 g.

7. Bacon and Eggs With Tomatoes

Preparation Time: 10 minutes.

Cooking Time: 30 minutes.

Servings: 5

Ingredients:

- 4 large ripe tomatoes, halved.
- 8 rashers smoked back bacon, trimmed of fat.
- 4 eggs.
- Salt to taste.
- Pepper to taste.
- 1 tsp. vinegar.

Directions:

1. Set up the grill to preheat. Let it preheat to high heat.
2. Place a rack on the grill pan. Line the pan with foil. Place tomatoes on the rack. Let it grill for 3 minutes. Place bacon along with the tomatoes.
3. Grill for 4 minutes until soft.
4. Meanwhile, place a large saucepan over medium-high heat. Fill the saucepan up to about ¾ with water. Let it boil.
5. When it begins to boil, add vinegar and stir. Crack an egg into a bowl and slowly slide the egg into the boiling water. Repeat this, one at a time.
6. Cook each egg until it is soft boiled, for 2–3 minutes.
7. Meanwhile, divide the bacon and tomatoes into 2 plates.
8. Remove the eggs with a slotted spoon and place them on the plates. Sprinkle salt and pepper and serve.

Nutrition:

- **Calories:** 110 g.
- **Fat:** 10 g.
- **Fiber:** 1 g.
- **Carbs:** 3 g.
- **Protein:** 6 g.

8. Cinnamon Porridge

Preparation Time: 10 minutes.

Cooking Time: 30 minutes.

Servings: 4

Ingredients:

- 4 ½ oz. jumbo porridge oats.
- 20 oz. semi-skimmed milk.
- 1 tsp. lemon juice.
- ½ tsp. ground cinnamon + extra to garnish.
- 2 ripe medium pears, peeled, cored, grated.

Directions:

1. Add oats, milk, and cinnamon into a nonstick saucepan. Place the saucepan over medium-low heat. Cook until creamy. Stir constantly.
2. Divide into bowls. Scatter pear on top. Drizzle lemon juice on top. Garnish with cinnamon and serve.

Nutrition:

- **Calories:** 383 g.
- **Fat:** 14 g.
- **Fiber:** 4 g.
- **Carbs:** 3 g.
- **Protein:** 8 g.

9. Cinnamon and Pecan Porridge

Preparation Time: 5 minutes.

Cooking Time: 10 minutes.

Servings: 2

Ingredients:

- ½ tsp. cinnamon.
- ¼ cup pecans, chopped.
- ¼ cup unsweetened coconut, toasted.
- ¼ cup coconut milk.
- ¼ cup almond butter.
- ¾ cup unsweetened almond milk.
- 1 tbsp. extra virgin coconut oil.
- 2 tbsps. hemp seeds.
- 2 tbsps. whole chia seeds.

Directions:

1. Place a small saucepan over medium heat. Combine the coconut milk, coconut oil, almond butter, and almond milk. Bring to simmer and remove from heat.
2. Add the toasted coconut (leave some for the topping), cinnamon, pecans, hemp seeds, and chia seeds. Mix the ingredients well and allow to rest for 5–10 minutes.
3. Divide between two bowls and serve.

Nutrition:

- **Calories:** 580 g.
- **Fat:** 14 g.
- **Fiber:** 10g.
- **Carbs:** 3 g.
- **Protein:** 8 g.

10. Sesame-Seared Salmon

Preparation Time: 5 minutes.

Cooking Time: 10 minutes.

Servings: 4

Ingredients:

- 4 wild salmon fillets (about 1lb.)
- 1 ½ tbsps. sesame seeds.
- 2 tbsps. toasted sesame oil.
- 1½ tbsps. avocado oil.
- 1 tsp. sea salt.

Directions:

1. Using a paper towel or a clean kitchen towel, pat the fillets to dry. Brush each with a tbsp. of sesame oil and season with a ½ tsp. of salt.
2. Place a large skillet over medium-high heat and drizzle with avocado oil. Once the oil is hot, add the salmon fillets with the flesh side down. Cook for about 3 minutes and flip. Cook the skin side for an additional 3–4 minutes, without overcooking it.
3. Remove the pan from the heat and brush with the remaining sesame oil. Season with the remaining salt and sprinkle with sesame seeds. Best served with a green salad.

Nutrition:

- **Calories:** 291 g.
- **Fat:** 14 g.
- **Fiber:** 6 g.
- **Carbs:** 3 g.
- **Protein:** 8 g.

11. Spring Ramen Bowl

Preparation Time: 15 minutes.

Cooking Time: 20 minutes.

Servings: 4

Ingredients:

- 3.53 oz. (100g) soba noodles.
- 4 eggs.
- 1 medium zucchini, julienned or grated.
- 4 cups chicken stock.
- 2 cups watercress.
- ½ cup snap peas.
- 1 cup mushrooms, finely sliced.
- 1 leek (white part only), finely sliced.
- 2 cloves garlic, minced.
- 1 long red chili, seeded and finely chopped.
- 1.6-inch ginger, minced.
- 1 tsp. sesame oil.
- 2 nori sheets, crumbled.
- 1 lemon, cut into wedges.
- 1 tbsp. olive oil.

Directions:

1. To boil the eggs, fill a saucepan with enough water to cover the eggs and set them over medium heat. Bring water to a gentle boil. Add the eggs and cook for 7 minutes. Drain and transfer the eggs into cold water. Set aside.
2. Place a medium-sized saucepan over medium-low heat. Heat the olive oil and sauté the garlic, ginger, leek, and chili for 5 minutes. Add the stock, noodles, and sesame oil. Cook for another 8 minutes or until noodles are cooked according to your desired doneness. During the last minute, add the zucchini, mushroom, and watercress.
3. Divide the ramen between four bowls and top with nori. Serve with eggs and lemon wedges.

Nutrition:

- **Calories:** 300 g.
- **Fat:** 12 g.
- **Fiber:** 1 g.
- **Carbs:** 3 g.
- **Protein:** 9 g.

12. Eggs and Salsa

Preparation Time: 5 minutes.

Cooking Time: 5 minutes.

Servings: 2

Ingredients:

- 3 cups tomatoes.
- 1 green onion (bunch).
- 1 bunch of cilantro, chopped.
- 1 cup red onion, chopped.
- Juice from 1 lime.
- 2 small habanero chilies, chopped.
- 2 garlic cloves, minced.
- 8 eggs, whisked.
- A drizzle of olive oil.
- Sea salt.

Directions:

1. Mix tomatoes, green onions, red onion, habaneros, garlic, cilantro, and lime juice and toss well.
2. Add a pinch of salt, toss again and keep this in the fridge until you serve it.
3. Heat up a pan with a drizzle of oil, add eggs, and scramble them for 4–5 minutes.
4. Divide scrambled eggs on plates, add salsa on top and serve.

Nutrition:

- **Calories:** 383 g.
- **Fat:** 14 g.
- **Fiber:** 4 g.
- **Carbs:** 3 g.
- **Protein:** 8 g.

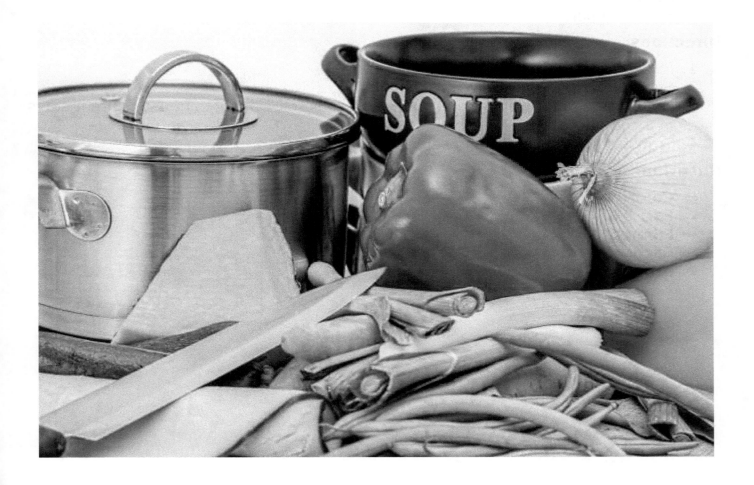

13. Poached Egg

Preparation Time: 5 minutes.

Cooking Time: 5 minutes.

Servings: 3

Ingredients:

- 1 tbsp. rice vinegar.
- 1 egg.
- Salt.
- Black pepper.

Directions:

1. Put some water into a pot and heat up.
2. Simmer gently, add vinegar, and whisk.
3. Crack the egg into simmering water and cook for 4 minutes making sure it stays in a compact shape.
4. Transfer egg to a plate and serve for breakfast.

Nutrition:

- **Calories:** 200 g.
- **Fat:** 8 g.
- **Fiber:** 2 g.
- **Carbs:** 8 g.
- **Protein:** 6 g.

14. Creamy Raspberry Cheesecake Bites

Preparation Time: 10 minutes.

Cooking Time: 30 minutes.

Servings: 4

Ingredients:

- ¾ cup butter.
- 6 drops of liquid stevia.
- 2 tsps. pure vanilla.
- $1/_8$ tsp. plus a pinch of sea salt, divided
- ¾ cup raw unsalted cashews.
- ¼ cup fresh raspberries halved (frozen berries work, just thaw and drain them well).
- ¼ cup raw unsalted pecans.
- $1/_8$ tsp ground cinnamon.

Directions:

1. Place the butter, stevia, vanilla, and $1/_8$ tsp. salt and blend. Pulse until the mixture is smooth. Scrape down the sides.
2. Add the cashews and process until nuts are broken down to the size of aquarium gravel or smaller.
3. Add the raspberries to a bowl. Stir them by hand and don't worry if some of them break while others stay whole. Cover and refrigerate for 30 minutes. The mixture will become firm.
4. Grind the pecans into a near flour-like state. Add cinnamon and salt.
5. Remove the batter from the refrigerator. Scoop out a tbsp. of the cheesecake mixture with a melon baller. While the batter is still in the melon baller, press the open end into the pecan dust. This is the flat side.
6. Release the batter with the flat side down on a plate. You have just made a cheesecake bite.
7. Before serving put it in the refrigerator for about an hour.

Nutrition:

- **Calories:** 33 g.
- **Fat:** 1 g.
- **Fiber:** 1 g.
- **Carbs:** 6 g.
- **Protein:** 2 g.

15. Decadent Cherry Chocolate Almond Clusters

Preparation Time: 10 minutes.

Cooking Time: 25 minutes.

Servings: 5

Ingredients:

- 1 tbsp. smooth nut butter of your choice.
- 8 oz. dark chocolate
- 1 cup oats.
- $1/3$ cup raw unsalted nuts, chopped.
- $1/3$ cup dried, unsweetened cherries or raisins, chopped.

Directions:

1. Boil water and simmer and then add the nut butter and chocolate, stirring occasionally for 2–3 minutes.
2. Take out from heat and stir in the oats, nuts, and dried fruit.
3. Stripe a baking sheet with wax or parchment paper.
4. Drib the batter by rounded teaspoonful onto the baking sheet, making 20 mounds.
5. Abode the baking sheet in the refrigerator for 25 minutes or until the mounds are set. Remove and store in an airtight container.

Nutrition:

- **Calories:** 260 g.
- **Fat:** 25 g.
- **Fiber:** 2 g.
- **Carbs:** 8 g.
- **Protein:** 2 g.

16. Low-Carb Waffles

Preparation Time: 10 minutes.

Cooking Time: 20 minutes.

Servings: 4

Ingredients:

- 6 eggs.
- 2 mashed bananas.
- 2 tsps. unsweetened almond butter.
- 3 tsps. quinoa flour.
- ¼ tsp. salt.
- ½ tsp. cinnamon powder.
- ½ tsp. olive oil extra virgin.
- ½ tbsp. coconut butter.
- ½ tbsp. almond butter.
- ¼ sliced banana.
- ½ tbsp. walnuts chopped.
- 1 tbsp. maple syrup.

Directions:

1. Plugin the waffle maker and let it heat up
2. Get a mixing container and in it mix the bananas mashed, eggs, quinoa flour, cinnamon, unsweetened almond butter, and salt until you get a smooth mixture.
3. When the waffle maker is hot enough, use the extra virgin olive oil to grease it.
4. Divide the waffle mixture into 3 portions and cook each until it is ready. Remove and do the same for the remaining mixture as well.
5. When cooled off, top the waffles with the remaining almond butter, quarter sliced bananas, and walnuts chopped maple syrup, and coconut butter.

Nutrition:

- **Calories:** 200 g.
- **Fat:** 8 g.
- **Fiber:** 2 g.
- **Carbs:** 8 g.
- **Protein:** 6 g.

17. Bacon Tacos

Preparation Time: 10 minutes.

Cooking Time: 20 minutes.

Servings: 4

Ingredients:

- 14 pieces halved bacon.
- 1 avocado seeded, peeled, and sliced.
- ¼ tsp. black pepper powder.
- ½ cup Monterey jack, shredded.
- 5 eggs.
- 2 tbsps. fresh chives chopped.
- 1 tbsp. almond milk
- A pinch of salt.
- 1 tbsp. unsweetened butter.
- A little hot sauce.

Directions:

1. Begin by preparing the taco shells first.
2. Heat the oven in advance at 400º c.
3. Get a baking sheet and line the inside with foil. Place the bacon strips in it, crisscrossing each other to form a square at the end. Do this again to form three consecutive weaves.
4. Take the black pepper powder and season the arranged bacon pieces and press flat the bacon using a baking rack that is inverted.
5. Place the sheet for baking in the oven that you heated in advance and let the bacon bake until it is crispy, which will take half an hour.
6. When the bacon is ready, using a knife for paring, cut up the crispy bacon squares to form small circles, which will be the taco shells. This should be done very fast.
7. Get the eggs and crack them in a mixing container. Add the almond milk and whisk both until they are well mixed.
8. Take a frying pan and over medium heat melt the unsweetened butter.
9. Follow this by pouring the whisked egg mixture and slowly move the eggs around to turn them into scrambled eggs. Add salt and black pepper powder for seasoning followed by chives then remove the frying pan from the heat.
10. Get a plate that you will use to serve and arrange the bacon taco shells on top of it.
11. Add the scrambled eggs on top of the bacon taco shells, then add a little cheese, avocado slices, and a little hot sauce as well.

Nutrition:

- **Calories:** 260 g. **Fat:** 8 g.
- **Fiber:** 2 g. **Carbs:** 8 g. **Protein:** 45 g.

18. Delicious Shakshuka

Preparation Time: 10 minutes.

Cooking Time: 30 minutes.

Servings: 4

Ingredients:

- ½ cup feta cheese crumbled.
- 2 tbsps. olive oil extra virgin
- 8 eggs.
- 1 onion sliced.
- 1 tsp. black pepper powder
- 1 large Red bell pepper, sliced.
- ¼ tsp. salt
- 3 garlic cloves, minced.
- ½ tsp. flakes of red pepper.
- 3 tomatoes blended.
- ½ tsp. coriander
- 2 tsps. cumin powder
- 1 tsp. paprika
- 1 tsp. fresh parsley chopped.
- 4 Pieces of almond bread for serving

Directions:

1. Heat your oven in advance at 375 º c.
2. Heat the olive oil in a large frying pan over medium heat.
3. Add the sliced onion and let it fry until it is a nice golden color. Top it off with the red bell pepper pieces and let this cook until the bell peppers are soft.
4. Add the minced garlic cloves to this mixture as well and let it cook until the garlic is nice and fragrant.
5. Add the sliced tomato, cumin powder, coriander, paprika, and flakes of red pepper. Also, add the salt and black pepper powder as well. Let this mix cook for 10 minutes until it thickens.
6. Get a large baking tin and pour in the cooked sauce. Using a spoon, create eight holes in the sauce and each crack an egg and pour it in.
7. Sprinkle a little salt and pepper over the eggs for seasoning. Using aluminum foil, cover the baking tin and transfer it into the oven you heated in advance for 15 minutes until the eggs are well cooked.
8. When they are ready, sprinkle the feta cheese that has been crumbled on top together with the fresh parsley as well.
9. Cut out slices and serve with the almond bread.

Nutrition:

- **Calories:** 122 g. **Fat:** 5.4 g.
- **Fiber:** 2 g. **Carbs:** 9.7 g.
- **Protein:** 8 g

19. Eggs With cauliflower

Preparation Time: 10 minutes.

Cooking Time: 20 minutes.

Servings: 4

Ingredients:

- ½ cauliflower head.
- 1 tbsp. olive oil extra virgin.
- 3 eggs.
- ¼ tsp. black pepper freshly ground.
- ¼ tsp. salt.
- ¼ tsp. cornstarch.
- 1 cup cheddar cheese shredded.
- 2 slices bacon.
- 2 tsps. paprika
- 1 tsp. fresh chives.

Directions:

1. Get a box grater, and with it, grate the half head of cauliflower until it is well grated.
2. Place the grated cauliflower into a mixing container and add an egg to it together with the cheddar cheese that has been shredded, cornstarch, and salt. Mix them all well.
3. Get a large frying pan and heat the olive oil over medium heat. Using a serving spoon, scoop the cauliflower mix into the frying pan and shape it into patties.
4. Cook these patties for five minutes until they are crispy and done. Ensure to flip both sides.
5. Get a saucepan and poach the remaining 2 eggs over medium heat using boiling water.
6. Get another pan for frying and over a medium flame, let the olive oil become hot. Follow this by adding in bacon pieces and allow them to cook until they are crispy.
7. Crack the eggs and remove them from the shell. Slice them into circles.
8. Place the cooked cauliflower patties on a plate and add the sliced eggs together with the slices of crispy bacon. Sprinkle the paprika and chives and serve.

Nutrition:

- **Calories:** 40 g.
- **Fat:** 1 g.
- **Fiber:** 2 g.
- **Carbs:** 8 g.
- **Protein:** 2 g.

20. Bacon With Brussels Sprouts and Eggs

Preparation Time: 20 minutes.

Cooking Time: 10 minutes.

Servings: 4

Ingredients:

- 6 eggs, large.
- 1 cup trimmed and halved brussels sprouts.
- ¼ tsp. black pepper freshly ground.
- 6 bacon slices.
- ¼ tsp. salt.
- 2 tbsps. olive oil extra virgin.
- 3 tbsps. buffalo sauce.
- ¼ tsp. flakes of red pepper.
- ½ tsp. powder of garlic.
- 1 tsp. fresh chives chopped.

Directions:

1. Heat your oven in advance at 425 º c.
2. Get a mixing container and in it mix the halved Brussels sprouts, powder of garlic, flakes of red pepper, bacon, buffalo sauce, and olive oil.
3. Add the black pepper that has been freshly ground and the salt to season the mix.
4. Get a large baking sheet and cover it with the mixture evenly.
5. Place the large baking sheet into the oven you heated in advance and let it bake for 15 minutes when the bacon will be crispy and the Brussels sprouts tender.
6. Take the sheet out and use a wooden spoon to make 6 holes in the baked mixture.
7. Crack the eggs and pour in the holes you made using the wooden spoon and sprinkle a little black pepper that has been freshly ground and salt to season the eggs.
8. Return the baking sheet into the oven and bake for 10 minutes until the eggs are done. Take the baking sheet out of the oven and sprinkle the fresh chives and buffalo sauce on top before serving.

Nutrition:

- **Calories:** 100 g.
- **Fat:** 7 g.
- Fiber: 2 g.
- **Carbs:** 8 g.
- **Protein:** 6 g.

21. Low Carb Bagels

Preparation Time: 10 minutes.

Cooking Time: 20 minutes.

Servings: 4

Ingredients:

- 2 cups almond flour
- 3 tbsps. bagel seasoning
- 1 tbsp. powder for baking
- 3 eggs.
- 3 cups mozzarella cheese, shredded.
- ¼ cup cream cheese.

Directions:

1. Heat your oven in advance at 400 º c.
2. Get 2 baking sheets and line them well with paper made from parchment.
3. Get a large mixing container and in it, mix the almond flour with the powder for baking.
4. Mix the mozzarella cheese and the cream cheese in a bowl that can be used in a microwave. Place the bowl in a microwave for 2 minutes when the cheese melts and combines.
5. Get the mixture of cheese from the bowl once out of the microwave and pour it into the mixing container with the flour from almonds and the powder for baking. Mix all the ingredients until well mixed.
6. Take the dough when done and divide it into eight parts that are equal in measure. Using your palms, take each of the eight dough parts and roll them into balls.
7. Using your fingers, create a hole in each of the balls, and gently stretch the dough to form the shape of a bagel.
8. Take one egg and beat it in a bowl. Brush the eggs on top of each made bagel following this by sprinkling the bagel seasoning at the top as well.
9. Place the bagel dough in the oven on its rack, which is in the middle for 25 minutes when they are nice and golden in color.
10.   Remove the bagels from the oven and let them get cold for about 10 minutes before serving them.

Nutrition:

- **Calories:** 275 g.
- **Fat:** 20 g.
- **Fiber:** 2 g.
- **Carbs:** 8 g.
- **Protein:** 20 g.

22. Healthy Breakfast Smoothie

Preparation Time: 5 minutes.

Cooking Time: 1 minute.

Servings: 1

Ingredients:

- 1 ¼ cups coconut milk, or almond or regular dairy milk.
- ½ cup kale or spinach, or both (¼ cup each) if you prefer.
- ½ avocado, sliced into smaller pieces.
- ¾ cup cucumber, cut into smaller pieces.
- 1 cup green grapes.
- ¼ tsp. ginger, peeled, and grated.
- 1 scoop plant-based protein powder.
- Honey, to taste.

Directions:

1. Orderly, mix all the ingredients in a small bowl.
2. Blend them until the mixture is smooth.
3. Taste the mixture and add as much honey as you desire.
4. Pour into a glass and serve.

Nutrition:

- **Calories:** 117 g.
- **Fats:** 15 g.
- **Protein:** 20 g.

23. Avocado-Egg Bowls

Preparation Time: 10 minutes.

Cooking Time: 40 minutes.

Servings: 3

Ingredients:

- 1 tsp. coconut oil.
- 2 organic eggs, free-range.
- Salt and pepper, to sprinkle.
- 1 avocado, large and ripe.

For garnishing:

- Chopped walnuts, as many as you like.
- Balsamic pearls, to taste.
- Fresh thyme, to taste.

Directions:

1. Slice the avocado in 2, then take out the pit and remove enough of the inside so that there is enough space inside to accommodate an entire egg.
2. Cut off a little bit of the bottom of the avocado so that the avocado will sit upright as you place it on a stable surface.
3. Open the eggs and put each of the yolks in a separate bowl or container. Place the egg whites in the same small bowl. Sprinkle some pepper and salt into the whites according to your taste, then mix them well.
4. Melt the coconut oil in a pan that has a lid that fits, and place it over medium-high heat.
5. Put the avocado "boats" meaty-side down and skin-side up in the pan, and sauté them for approx. 35 seconds, or when they become darker.
6. Turn them over, then add to the spaces inside, almost filling the inside with the egg whites.
7. Then lower the temperature and cover the pan. Let them sit covered for approx. 16–20 minutes, or until the whites are just about fully cooked.
8. Gently, add 1 yolk onto each of the avocados and keep cooking them for 4–5 minutes, or just until they get to the point of cooking you want them to.
9. Move the avocados to a dish and add toppings to each of them using the walnuts, the balsamic pearls, or/and thyme.

Nutrition:

- **Calories:** 215 g.
- **Fats:** 18 g.
- **Protein:** 9 g.

24. Blueberries Breakfast Bowl

Preparation Time: 35 minutes.

Cooking Time: 0 minutes.

Servings: 1

Ingredients:

- 1 tsp. chia seed.
- 1 cup almond milk.
- ¼ cup fresh blueberries or fresh fruits.

Directions:

1. Mix the chia seeds with almond milk. Stir periodically.
2. Put in the fridge to cool and serve with the blueberries or fresh fruit. Enjoy!

Nutrition:

- **Calories:** 202 g.
- **Fats:** 16.8 g.
- **Protein:** 10.2 g.

25. Feta-Filled Tomato-Topped Oldie Omelet

Preparation Time: 5 minutes.

Cooking Time: 6 minutes.

Servings: 1

Ingredients:

- 1 tbsp. coconut oil.
- 2 eggs.
- 1 ½ tbsps. milk.
- A dash of salt and pepper.
- ¼ cup tomatoes, sliced into cubes.
- 2 tbsps. feta cheese, crumbled.

Directions:

1. Beat the eggs with pepper, salt, milk, and the remaining spices.
2. Pour the mixture along with coconut oil into a preheated pan.
3. Stir in the tomatoes and cheese. Cook for 6 minutes, or until the cheese melts.

Nutrition:

- **Calories:** 335 g.
- **Fats:** 28.4 g.
- **Protein:** 16.2 g.

26. Carrot Breakfast Salad

Cooking Time: 4 hours.

Preparation Time: 5 minutes.

Servings: 4

Ingredients:

- 2 tbsps. olive oil.
- 2 lbs. baby carrots, peeled and halved.
- 3 garlic cloves, minced.
- 2 yellow onions, chopped.
- ½ cup vegetable stock.
- $^1/_3$ cup tomatoes, crushed.
- A pinch of salt and black pepper.

Directions:

1. In your slow cooker, combine all the ingredients, cover, and cook on high for 4 hours.
2. Divide into bowls and serve for breakfast.

Nutrition:

- **Calories:** 437 g.
- **Protein:** 2.39 g.
- **Fats:** 39.14 g.

27. Paprika Lamb Chops

Preparation Time: 10 minutes.

Cooking Time: 15 minutes.

Servings: 4

Ingredients:

- 2 lamb racks, cut into chops.
- Salt and pepper, to taste.
- 3 tbsps. paprika.
- ¾ cup cumin powder.
- 1 tsp. chili powder.

Directions:

1. Take a bowl and add the paprika, cumin, chili, salt, pepper, and stir.
2. Add the lamb chops and rub the mixture.
3. Heat grill over medium heat, add the lamb chops, and cook for 5 minutes.
4. Flip the lamb chops over and cook for 5 minutes more, then flip again.
5. Cook for 2 minutes, flip, and cook for 2 minutes more. Serve and enjoy.

Nutrition:

- **Calories:** 200 g.
- **Fats:** 5 g.
- **Protein:** 8 g.

28. Delicious Turkey Wrap

Preparation Time: 10 minutes.

Cooking Time: 10 minutes.

Servings: 6

Ingredients:

- 1 ¼ lb. ground turkey, lean.
- 4 green onions, minced.
- 1 tbsp. olive oil.
- 1 garlic clove, minced.
- 2 tsps. chili paste.
- 8 oz. water chestnut, diced.
- 3 tbsps. hoisin sauce.
- 2 tbsps. coconut amino.
- 1 tbsp. rice vinegar.
- 12 butter lettuce leaves.
- $\frac{1}{8}$ tsp. salt.

Directions:

1. Take a pan and place it over medium heat, then add the turkey, and garlic to the pan.
2. Heat for 6 minutes, or until cooked.
3. Transfer the turkey to a bowl.
4. Add the onions and water chestnuts.
5. Stir in the hoisin sauce, coconut amino, rice vinegar, and chili paste.
6. Toss well and transfer the mix to the lettuce leaves. Serve and enjoy.

Nutrition:

- **Calories:** 162 g.
- **Fats:** 4 g.
- **Protein:** 23 g.

29. Bacon & Chicken Garlic Wrap

Preparation Time: 15 minutes.

Cooking Time: 10 minutes.

Servings: 4

Ingredients:

- 1 chicken fillet, cut into small cubes.
- 8–9 bacon slices, thinly cut to fit the cubes. dx
- 6 garlic cloves, minced

Directions: {7

1. Preheat your oven to 400º F.
2. Line a baking tray with aluminum foil.
3. Add the minced garlic to a bowl and rub each chicken piece with it.
4. Wrap a bacon piece around each garlic chicken bite.
5. Secure each bite with a toothpick.
6. Transfer the bites to the baking sheet, keeping a little bit of space between them.
7. Bake for about 15–20 minutes, or until crispy. Serve and enjoy.

Nutrition:

- **Calories:** 260 g.
- **Fats:** 19 g.
- **Protein:** 22 g.

30. Pumpkin Pancakes

Preparation Time: 10 minutes.

Cooking Time: 15 minutes.

Servings: 6

Ingredients:

- 3 eggs, large, and egg whites separated.
- $^2/_3$ cups organic oats.
- 6 oz. pumpkin purée.
- 1 scoop collagen peptides.
- 1 tsp. stevia powder.
- ½ tsp. cinnamon.
- Cooking spray, as needed.
- Fruits (optional).

Directions:

1. Combine and blend all the ingredients in a blender and mix well.
2. Apply the cooking spray to the pan to coat it properly.
3. Pour some of the batter into the pan to coat the pan properly.
4. Wait till the edges of the pancake brown up a little bit.
5. Flip the pancake over and cook from the other side.
6. You can serve it with fruits.

Nutrition:

- **Calories:** 70 g.
- **Fats:** 3 g.
- **Protein:** 3 g.

31. Cherry Smoothie Bowl

Preparation Time: 15 minutes.

Cooking Time: 0 minutes.

Servings: 1

Ingredients:

- ½ cup organic rolled oats.
- ½ cup almond milk, unsweetened.
- 1 tbsp. chia seeds.
- 1 tsp. hemp seeds.
- 2 tsps. almonds, sliced.
- 1 tbsp. almond butter.
- 1 tsp. vanilla extract.
- ½ cup berries, fresh.
- 1 cup cherries, frozen.
- 1 cup plain Greek yogurt.

Directions:

1. Soak the organic rolled oats in almond milk.
2. Prepare a smooth blend with the soaked oats, frozen cherries, yogurt, chia seeds, almond butter, and vanilla extract. Pour the mixture into 2 bowls.
3. To each bowl, add equal parts of the hemp seeds, sliced almonds, and fresh cherries.

Nutrition:

- **Calories:** 130 g.
- **Fats:** 0 g.
- **Protein:** 1 g.

32. Kale & Sausage Omelet

Preparation Time: 10 minutes.

Cooking Time: 10 minutes.

Servings: 2

Ingredients:

- 4 eggs.
- 2 cups kale, chopped.
- 4 oz. sausages, sliced.
- 4 tbsps. ricotta cheese.
- 6 oz. roasted squash.
- 2 tbsps. olive oil.
- Salt and black pepper, to taste.
- Fresh parsley, for garnishing.

Directions:

1. In a medium-sized bowl, blend the eggs, salt, and pepper. Then whisk in the kale and the ricotta cheese. In another bowl, mash the squash.
2. Add the squash to the egg mixture. In a pan over medium heat, heat 1 tbsp. of olive oil and cook the sausages for 5 minutes. Drizzle the remaining olive oil.
3. Pour the egg mixture over and cook for 2 minutes on both sides. With a spatula, run around the edges of the omelet and slide it onto a platter. Serve topped with parsley.

Nutrition:

- **Calories:** 258 g.
- **Fats:** 22 g.
- **Protein:** 12 g.

33. Sausage Quiche With Tomatoes

Preparation Time: 15 minutes.

Cooking Time: 10 minutes.

Servings: 6

Ingredients:

- 6 eggs
- 12 oz. raw sausage rolls.
- 10 cherry tomatoes halved.
- 2 tbsps. heavy cream.
- 2 tbsps. Parmesan, grated.
- Salt and black pepper, to taste.
- 2 tbsps. parsley, chopped.
- 5 eggplant slices.

Directions:

1. Preheat the oven to 370º F. Press the sausage rolls onto the bottom of a greased pie dish. On top of the sausage, carefully arrange the eggplant slices.
2. Top with cherry tomatoes. Whisk together the eggs along with the heavy cream, Parmesan cheese, salt, and pepper.
3. Spoon the egg mixture over the sausage and bake for about 40 minutes. Serve with parsley.

Nutrition:

- **Calories:** 340 g.
- **Fats:** 28 g.
- **Protein:** 1.7 g.

34. Bacon & Cream Cheese Mug Muffins

Preparation Time: 15 minutes.

Cooking Time: 15 minutes.

Servings: 2

Ingredients:

- ¼ cup flaxseed meal.
- 1 egg.
- 2 tbsps. heavy cream.
- 2 tbsps. pesto.
- ¼ cup almond flour.
- ¼ tsp. baking soda.
- Salt and black pepper, to taste.
- 2 tbsps. cream cheese.
- 4 bacon slices.
- ½ medium avocado, sliced.

Directions:

1. Mix the flaxseed meal, almond flour, and baking soda in a bowl. Add the egg, heavy cream, and pesto. Then whisk well. Season with salt and pepper.
2. Divide the mixture between 2 ramekins. Microwave for 60–90 seconds. Let cool slightly before filling.
3. Put the bacon in a nonstick skillet and cook until crispy, then set aside.
4. Transfer the muffins onto a plate and cut them in half crosswise. Assemble the sandwiches by spreading the cream cheese and topping with the bacon and avocado slices.

Nutrition:

- **Calories:** 511 g.
- **Fats:** 38 g.
- **Protein:** 16 g.

35. Chorizo & Cheese Omelet

Preparation Time: 10 minutes.

Cooking Time: 10 minutes.

Servings: 2

Ingredients:

- 4 eggs, beaten
- 4 oz. mozzarella, grated
- 1 tbsp. butter
- 8 chorizo slices, thin
- 1 tomato, sliced
- Salt and black pepper to taste

Directions:

1. Whisk the eggs with salt and pepper.
2. In a cast-iron skillet, add the butter and cook the eggs for 30 seconds. Create a layer with the chorizo slices.
3. Arrange the sliced tomato and mozzarella over the chorizo and cook for about 3 minutes. Cover the skillet and continue cooking for 3 more minutes, or until the omelet is completely set.
4. With a spatula, run around the edges of the omelet and flip it onto a plate folded-side down. Serve.

Nutrition:

- **Calories:** 451 g.
- **Fats:** 36.5 g.
- **Protein:** 30 g.

Lunch

36. Soy Lime Roasted Tofu

Preparation Time: 15 minutes.

Cooking Time: 1 hour 35 minutes.

Servings: 4

Ingredients:

- 28 oz. extra-firm tofu, drained and cubed.
- $2/3$ cup reduced-sodium soy sauce.
- $2/3$ cup lime juice.
- 6 tbsps. sesame oil, toasted.

Directions:

1. In a bowl, mix oil, lime juice, and sauce. Toss in tofu. Refrigerate for 1 hour to marinate.
2. Set oven to 450º F
3. Remove tofu from marinade and spread on 2 baking sheets with some spacing between the pieces. Roast for 20 minutes as you turn halfway until golden brown.

Nutrition:

- **Calories:** 163.
- **Fat:** 11 g.
- **Carbs:** 2 g.
- **Protein:** 19 g.

37. Chicken Nuggets

Preparation Time: 5 minutes.

Cooking Time: 20 minutes.

Servings: 6

Ingredients:

- 2 cups chicken, cooked.
- 8 oz. cream cheese.
- 1 egg.
- ¼ cup almond flour.
- 1 tsp. garlic salt.

Directions:

1. While the chicken is still warm, set it in an electric mixer and shred. In case you are using leftover chicken, warm it up for a short time.
2. Once the shredding is done, add all the remaining ingredients and mix it up.
3. Drop scoops of the mixture onto a greased baking sheet, flatten it into a nugget shape.
4. Bake it for 13 minutes at 350º F, till they turn golden and cooked.
5. Enjoy when hot!

Nutrition:

- **Calories:** 150 g.
- **Fat:** 18 g.
- **Protein:** 15 g.
- **Carbs:** 1.8 g.

38. Crab-Stuffed Avocado

Preparation Time: 10 minutes.

Cooking Time: 5 minutes.

Servings: 5

Ingredients:

- 1 lb. crab.
- 1 avocado, ripe, pitted, peeled.
- 2 tbsps. onion, finely chopped.
- 2 tbsps. cilantro, chopped.
- Salt.
- Pepper.

Directions:

1. Place the crab in the Instant Pot and add a cup of water.
2. Set the lid in place and the vent should point to "Sealing."
3. Set the IP to manual and cook for 5 minutes.
4. Do quick pressure release.
5. Take the crab out and let it cool.
6. Extract the meat from the crab and discard the shells.
7. In a bowl, combine the crabmeat and stir in the rest of the ingredients.
8. Refrigerate.
9. Serve chilled.

Nutrition:

- **Calories:** 149 g.
- **Carbs:** 4.7 g.
- **Protein:** 13.2 g.
- **Fat:** 15.3 g.

39. Thai Fish Curry

Preparation Time: 5 minutes.

Cooking Time: 10 minutes.

Servings: 6

Ingredients:

- $1/3$ cup olive oil.
- 1 ½ lb. salmon fillets.
- 2 cups coconut milk, freshly squeezed.
- 2 tbsps. curry powder.
- ¼ cup cilantro chopped.

Directions:

1. In your instant pot, add in all ingredients. Apply a seasoning of pepper and salt.
2. Give a good stir.
3. Set the lid in place and the vent to point to "Sealing."
4. Set the IP to "Manual" and cook for 10 minutes.
5. Do quick pressure release.

Nutrition:

- **Calories:** 470 g.
- **Carbs:** 5.6 g.
- **Protein:** 25.5 g.
- **Fat:** 39.8 g.

40. Avocado Grapefruit Salad

Preparation Time: 5 minutes.

Cooking Time: 20 minutes.

Servings: 4

Ingredients:

- 2 avocados, peeled, pitted and meat scooped.
- 1 grapefruit, red, peeled.
- ¼ cup pomegranate seeds.
- 1 tbsp. shallots, minced.
- ¼ cup olive oil.
- 1 tbsp. pomegranate juice.
- Salt.
- Pepper.

Directions:

1. Squeeze some of the grapefruit to obtain the juice. Sprinkle over the avocados in a bowl. Spread over the remaining grapefruit and the pomegranate seeds.
2. In another bowl, mix olive oil, salt, pepper, pomegranate juice, and shallots. Sprinkle over the salad and enjoy.

Nutrition:

- **Calories:** 335 g.
- **Fat:** 18 g.
- **Protein:** 3 g.
- **Carbs:** 28 g.

41. BBQ Pork Tenders

Preparation Time: 15 minutes.

Cooking Time: 7 minutes.

Servings: 4

Ingredients:

- 1 tsp. Erythritol.
- 3 tbsps. ground paprika.
- 1 tsp. ground black pepper.
- 1 tsp. salt.
- ½ tsp. chili powder.
- ¼ tsp. cayenne pepper.
- 1 tsp. garlic powder.
- 14 oz. pork loins.
- 1 tbsp. olive oil.
- 1 tbsp. almond butter.

Directions:

1. Make the BBQ mix: in the shallow bowl, mix up together ground paprika, Erythritol, ground black pepper, salt, chili powder, cayenne pepper, garlic powder.
2. Cut the pork loin into the tenders.
3. Rub every pork loin with BBQ mix and sprinkle with olive oil.
4. Leave the meat to marinate for at least 15 minutes.
5. After this, place almond butter in the skillet and melt it.
6. Place the pork tenders in the almond butter and cook them for 5 minutes.
7. Then flip the meat onto another side and cook for 2 minutes more. The time of cooking depends on meat thickness.

Nutrition:

- **Calories:** 315 g.
- **Fat:** 20.3 g.
- **Fiber:** 2.7 g.
- **Carbs:** 4.7 g.
- **Protein:** 29 g.

42. Fish Bars

Preparation Time: 10 minutes.

Cooking Time: 15 minutes.

Servings: 6

Ingredients:

- 10 oz. tilapia fillet.
- ½ cup coconut flour.
- 2 eggs, whisked.
- 1 tsp. salt.
- ½ tsp. ground black pepper.
- 3 oz. Parmesan, grated.
- 1 tsp. butter.

Directions:

1. Mince the tilapia fillet and place it in the mixing bowl.
2. Add coconut flour, whisked eggs, salt, ground black pepper, and grated cheese.
3. Mix up the mixture with the help of the spoon until homogenous.
4. Spread the casserole mold with the butter generously.
5. Place the fish mixture in the mold and flatten it well. Cut the mixture into the bars with the help of the knife.
6. Preheat the oven to 360° F.
7. Place the casserole mold in the oven and cook the fish bars for 15 minutes or until the fish bars get the golden-brown surface.
8. Chill the cooked meal well and only after this, transfer it to the serving plates.

Nutrition:

- **Calories:** 128 g.
- **Fat:** 5.8 g.
- **Fiber:** 0.5 g.
- **Carbs:** 1.4 g.
- **Protein:** 17.6 g.

43. Pan-Fried Cod

Preparation Time: 5 minutes.

Cooking Time: 10 minutes.

Servings: 2

Ingredients:

- 12 oz. cod fillet.
- 1 tbsp. scallions, chopped.
- 1 tbsp. butter.
- 1 tbsp. coconut oil.
- 1 tsp. garlic, diced.
- 1 tsp. cumin seeds.
- 1 tsp. coriander seeds.
- 1 tsp. salt.

Directions:

1. Place butter and coconut oil in the skillet and melt them.
2. Add garlic, scallions, cumin, and coriander seeds.
3. Rub the fish fillet with salt and place it in the skillet.
4. Fry the fish for 2 minutes from each side or until it is light brown.
5. Transfer the cooked cod fillet to the plate and cut into 2 servings.

Nutrition:

- **Calories:** 253 g.
- **Fat:** 14.3 g.
- **Fiber:** 0.2 g.
- **Carbs:** 1.2 g.
- **Protein:** 30.8 g.

44. Orange and Garlic Shrimp

Preparation Time: 20 minutes.

Cooking Time: 10 minutes.

Servings: 6

Ingredients:

- 1 large orange.
- 3 tbsps. extra-virgin olive oil, divided.
- 1 tbsp. chopped fresh rosemary (about 3 sprigs) or 1 tsp. dried rosemary.
- 1 tbsp. chopped fresh thyme (about 6 sprigs) or 1 tsp. dried thyme.
- 3 garlic cloves, minced (about 1 ½ tsp.)
- ¼ tsp. freshly ground black pepper.
- ¼ tsp. kosher or sea salt.
- 1 ½ lbs. fresh raw shrimp, (or frozen and thawed raw shrimp) shells and tails removed.

Directions:

1. Zest the entire orange using a Microplane or citrus grater.
2. In a large zip-top plastic bag, combine the orange zest and 2 tbsps. of oil with rosemary, thyme, garlic, pepper, and salt.
3. Add the shrimp, seal the bag, and gently massage the shrimp until all the ingredients are combined and the shrimp is completely covered with the seasonings. Set aside.
4. Heat a grill, grill pan, or a large skillet over medium heat.
5. Brush on or swirl in the remaining 1 tbsp. of oil. Add half the shrimp, and cook for 4 to 6 minutes, or until the shrimp turn pink and white, flipping halfway through if on the grill or stirring every minute if in a pan.
6. Transfer the shrimp to a large serving bowl. Repeat with the remaining shrimp, and add them to the bowl.
7. While the shrimp cook, peel the orange and cut the flesh into bite-size pieces. Add to the serving bowl, and toss with the cooked shrimp. Serve immediately or refrigerate and serve cold.

Nutrition:

- **Calories:** 170 g.
- **Fat:** 8 g.
- **Fiber:** 1 g.
- **Carbs:** 5 g.
- **Protein:** 24 g.

45. Chicken Lentil Stew

Preparation Time: 10 minutes.

Cooking Time: 25 minutes.

Servings: 6

Ingredients:

- 2 lbs. chicken thighs, boneless & skinless.
- 1 tbsp. olive oil.
- 1 cup onion, chopped.
- 4 cups chicken stock.
- 8 oz. green lentils, soak for 1 hour.
- 28 oz. can tomato, diced.
- Pepper.
- Salt.

Directions:

1. Add oil into the inner pot of Instant Pot and set the pot on sauté mode.
2. Add onion and sauté for 5 minutes.
3. Add the rest of the ingredients and stir well.
4. Seal pot with lid and cook on high for minutes.
5. Once done, release pressure using quick release. Remove lid.
6. Shred chicken using a fork.
7. Stir well and serve.

Nutrition:

- **Calories:** 479 g.
- **Fat:** 14 g.
- **Fiber:** 4 g.
- **Carbs:** 30 g.
- **Protein:** 55 g.

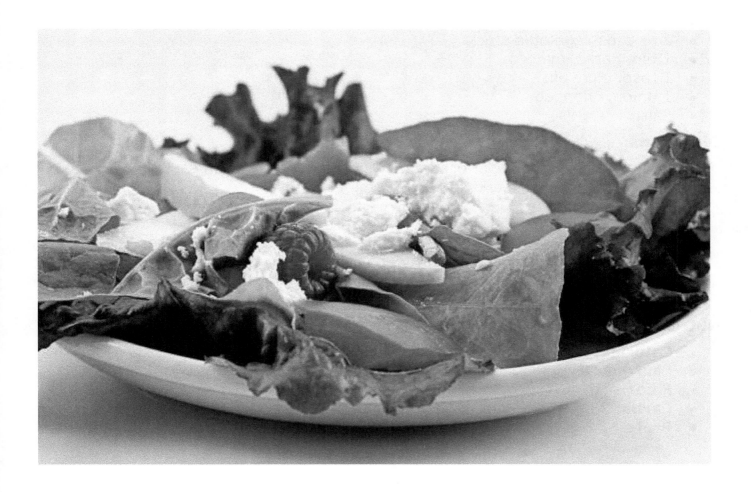

46. Garlic Squash Broccoli Soup

Preparation Time: 10 minutes.

Cooking Time: 15 minutes.

Servings: 4

Ingredients:

- 1 lb. butternut squash, peeled and diced.
- 1 lb. broccoli florets.
- 1 tsp. dried basil.
- 1 tsp. paprika.
- 2 ½ cups vegetable stock.
- 1 tsp. garlic, minced.
- 1 tbsp. olive oil.
- 1 onion, chopped.
- Salt.

Directions:

1. Add oil into the inner pot of Instant Pot and set the pot on sauté mode.
2. Add onion and garlic and sauté for 3 minutes.
3. Add remaining ingredients and stir well.
4. Seal pot with lid and cook on high pressure 12 for minutes.
5. Once done, allow to release pressure naturally for 10 minutes then release remaining using quick release. Remove lid.
6. Blend soup using an immersion blender until smooth.
7. Serve and enjoy.

Nutrition:

- **Calories:** 70 g.
- **Fat:** 4 g.
- **Fiber:** 4 g.
- **Carbs:** 30 g.
- **Protein:** 2 g.

47. Lamb Curry

Preparation Time: 10 minutes.

Cooking Time: 4 hours.

Servings: 6

Ingredients:

- 2 tbsps. fresh ginger, grated.
- 2 garlic cloves, peeled and minced.
- 2 tsps. cardamom.
- 1 onion, peeled, and chopped.
- 6 cloves.
- 1 lb. lamb meat, cubed.
- 2 tsps. cumin powder.
- 1 tsp. garam masala.
- ½ tsp. chili powder.
- 1 tsp. turmeric.
- 2 tsps. coriander.
- 1 lb. spinach.
- 14 oz. tomatoes, canned.

Directions:

1. In a slow cooker, mix lamb with tomatoes, spinach, ginger, garlic, onion, cardamom, cloves, cumin, garam masala, chili, turmeric, and coriander.
2. Stir well. Cover and cook on high for 4 hours.
3. Uncover slow cooker, stir the chili, divide into bowls, and serve.

Nutrition:

- **Calories:** 186 g.
- **Fat:** 7 g.
- **Fiber:** 2 g.
- **Carbs:** 8 g.
- **Protein:** 26 g.

48. Healthy Baby Carrots

Preparation Time: 10 minutes.

Cooking Time: 20 minutes.

Servings: 4

Ingredients:

- 1 lb. baby carrots.
- 1 tsp. Italian seasoning.
- 1 tbsp. balsamic vinegar.
- 2 tbsps. olive oil.
- ¼ cup vegetable stock.
- Pepper.
- Salt.

Directions:

1. Add all ingredients into the inner pot of the Instant Pot and stir well.
2. Seal pot with lid and cook on high for 20 minutes.
3. Once done, allow to release pressure naturally for 5 minutes then release remaining using quick release. Remove lid.
4. Serve and enjoy.

Nutrition:

- **Calories:** 105 g.
- **Fat:** 7.5 g.
- **Carbs:** 9.6 g.
- **Protein:** 0.8 g.

49. Garlic Mushrooms Lamb Chops

Preparation Time: 10 minutes.

Cooking Time: 15 minutes.

Servings: 4

Ingredients:

- 1 lb. lamb chops.
- 2 cups beef stock.
- 1 cup mushrooms, sliced.
- 2 tbsps. olive oil.
- 1 tsp. garlic, minced.
- Pepper.
- Salt.

Directions:

1. Add all ingredients into the inner pot of the Instant Pot and stir well.
2. Seal pot with lid and cook on high for 15 minutes.
3. Once done, release pressure using quick release. Remove lid.
4. Stir and serve.

Nutrition:

- **Calories:** 284 g.
- **Fat:** 15.6 g.
- **Carbs:** 0.9 g.
- **Protein:** 33.8 g.

50. Eggplant & Lamb

Preparation Time: 10 minutes.

Cooking Time: 35 minutes.

Servings: 4

Ingredients:

- 2 lamb shanks.
- 1 bay leaf.
- 2 tbsps. cumin seeds.
- 1 tbsp. oregano.
- ½ eggplant, cubed.
- ¼ cup yogurt.
- 4 cups beef broth.
- 2 tbsps. olive oil.
- 1 tbsp. garlic, minced.
- 2 green chilies, chopped.
- Pepper.
- Salt.

Directions:

1. Add oil into the inner pot of Instant Pot and set the pot on sauté mode.
2. Add cumin, oregano, garlic, pepper, and salt and sauté for 2 minutes.
3. Add meat and sauté for 3 minutes.
4. Add eggplant and cook for 5 minutes.
5. Add remaining ingredients and stir well.
6. Seal pot with lid and cook on high for 30 minutes.
7. Once done, release pressure using quick release. Remove lid.
8. Stir and serve.

Nutrition:

- **Calories:** 452 g.
- **Fat:** 23 g.
- **Fiber:** 4 g.
- **Carbs:** 9 g.
- **Protein:** 53 g.

51. Asian Chicken Wings

Preparation Time: 10 minutes.

Cooking Time: 35 minutes.

Servings: 5

Ingredients:

- 2 lbs. chicken wings.
- 2 tbsps. sesame oil.
- ¼ cup tamari sauce.
- 1 tbsp. ginger powder.
- 2 tsps. white wine vinegar.
- 3 garlic cloves, minced.
- ¼ tsp. sea salt.

Directions:

1. Preheat oven to 400º F.
2. In a large container, whisk together the ginger powder, sesame oil, salt, tamari sauce, vinegar, and garlic.
3. Add the wings to the mixture and stir to coat.
4. Place the wings on a lined baking sheet and bake for 30–35 minutes until golden and crispy.
5. If you want it crispier, turn on the broiler for a few minutes. Enjoy!

Nutrition:

- **Calories:** 277 g.
- **Carbs:** 1 g.
- **Fats:** 22 g.
- **Protein:** 18 g.

52. Bok Choy Samba

Preparation Time: 5 minutes.

Cooking Time: 15 minutes.

Servings: 3

Ingredients:

- 1 onion sliced.
- 4 bok choy, sliced.
- 4 tbsps. coconut cream.
- Salt and freshly ground black pepper, to taste.
- ½ cup parmesan cheese, grated.

Directions:

1. Start by tossing the bok choy with salt and black pepper for seasoning.
2. Add oil to any large-sized pan and sauté the onion in it for 5 minutes.
3. Stir in the bok choy and coconut cream. Stir-cook for 6 minutes.
4. Toss in the cheese and cover the skillet to cook over low heat for 3 minutes. Enjoy fresh and warm.

Nutrition:

- **Calories:** 112 g.
- **Fats:** 4.9 g.
- **Saturated Fats:** 1.9 g.
- **Cholesterol:** 10 mg.
- **Sodium:** 355 mg.
- **Carbs:** 1.9 g.
- **Sugar:** 0.8 g.
- **Fiber:** 0.4 g.
- **Protein:** 3 g.

53. Pimiento Cheese Meatballs

Preparation Time: 30 minutes.

Cooking Time: 20 minutes.

Servings: 4

Ingredients:

- $^1/_3$ cup mayonnaise.
- ¼ cup pimientos or pickled jalapeños.
- 1 tsp. chili or paprika powder.
- 1 tbsp. Dijon mustard.
- 1 pinch cayenne pepper.
- 4 oz. grated cheddar cheese.

For the meatballs:

- 1 ½ lb. ground beef.
- 1 egg.
- 2 tbsps. butter for frying.
- Salt and pepper.

Directions:

1. In a large bowl, mix all the ingredients for the pimiento cheese.
2. Add the egg and some ground beef to the cheese mixture. To mix the ingredients, you may need a wooden spoon, or use your hands. We recommend using latex gloves when handling raw meat. Add salt and pepper to taste.
3. Once you've used the mixture to form large meatballs, fry them in butter in a pan over medium heat until they are cooked thoroughly. Use a side dish of your choice (some cooked vegetables would be a great choice) and perhaps serve it with a green salad and homemade mayonnaise.
4. This recipe is for 4 servings and the meal only has 1 gram of carbs (not including the side dish).

Nutrition:

- **Calories:** 660 g.
- **Fats:** 53 g.
- **Carbs:** 1 g.
- **Protein:** 42 g.

54. Bacon-Wrapped Salmon

Preparation Time: 10 minutes.

Cooking Time: 20 minutes.

Servings: 2

Ingredients:

- 2 salmon fillets.
- 1 tbsp. olive oil.
- 4 slices bacon.
- Lemon wedges.
- 2 tbsps. tarragon.

Directions:

1. Preheat the oven to 350º F.
2. Pat the fillets dry.
3. Wrap the bacon around the salmon fillets.
4. Place fillets on a roasting tray and drizzle with olive oil.
5. Bake for 15–20 minutes.
6. Garnish with lemon wedges and chopped tarragon.

Nutrition:

- **Calories:** 612 g.
- **Carbs:** 7.1 g.
- **Fats:** 42 g.
- **Protein:** 53.3 g.

55. Slow Cooker Bacon and Chicken

Preparation Time: 5 minutes.

Cooking Time: 8 hours.

Servings: 4

Ingredients:

- 5 chicken breasts.
- 10 slices bacon.
- 2 tbsps. thyme, dried.
- 1 tbsp. oregano, dried.
- 1 tbsp. rosemary, dried.
- 5 tbsps. olive oil, divided.
- 1 tbsp. salt.

Directions:

1. In a slow cooker pot, mix all the ingredients and 2 tbsps. of olive oil.
2. Cook on low for 8 hours.
3. Shred the meat and mix with the remaining olive oil.

Nutrition:

- **Calories:** 315 g.
- **Carbs:** 3.6 g.
- **Fats:** 24 g.
- **Protein:** 22.9 g.

56. Aromatic Dover Sole Fillets

Preparation Time: 5 minutes.

Cooking Time: 20 minutes.

Servings: 2

Ingredients:

- 6 Dover sole fillets.
- ¼ cup virgin olive oil.
- 1 lemon zested.
- A dash of cardamom powder.
- 1 cup fresh cilantro leaves.
- Pinch of sea salt.

Directions:

1. Bring the fillets to room temperature.
2. Set the oven's broiler to "high."
3. Pour ½ of the oil into an oven tray.
4. Add ½ of the cilantro leaves, half of the lemon zest, and the cardamom powder.
5. Lay the fillets in the mixture and top with the remaining ingredients.
6. Set under the broiler for about 7–8 minutes, or until the fish breaks easily with a fork and it is not transparent.
7. Serve immediately.

Nutrition:

- **Calories:** 244 g.
- **Carbs:** 2.9 g.
- **Fats:** 17.9 g.
- **Protein:** 18.6 g.

57. Chicken and Prosciutto Spiedini

Preparation Time: 15 minutes.

Cooking Time: 10 minutes.

Servings: 8

Ingredients:

- 8 raw chicken tenders.
- 8 oz. block provolone cheese.
- 8 slices prosciutto.
- ½ tsp. kosher salt.
- $\frac{1}{8}$ tsp. ground black pepper.
- 16 fresh basil leaves.
- ¼ tsp. garlic powder.
- 8 skewers.

Directions:

1. Combine the garlic powder, kosher salt, and pepper.
2. Cut the chicken tenders off the tendons, cutting them into ½-inch pieces.
3. Season the chicken with the spice mixture.
4. Cut the provolone cheese into pieces about 1–2 inches long.
5. On a cutting board, place a slice of prosciutto. Then top with 1 chicken tender and 2 leaves of fresh basil. Next place 1 piece of cheese across the basil.
6. Carefully, roll the bundle and skewer it.
7. Preheat a grill to 325–375º F. Grill for about 3–5 minutes per side, or until a thermometer reads 165º F in the center and the skewers are cooked through.
8. Serve warm.

Nutrition:

- **Calories:** 174 g.
- **Carbs:** 0.75 g.
- **Fats:** 10 g.
- **Protein:** 20 g.

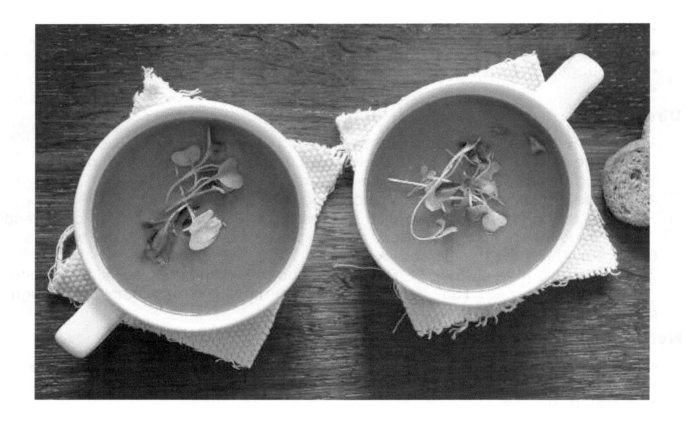

58. Lemon Baked Salmon

Preparation Time: 5 minutes.

Cooking Time: 20 minutes.

Servings: 2

Ingredients:

- 12 oz. salmon fillets.
- 2 lemons, sliced thinly.
- 2 tbsps. olive oil.
- Salt and black pepper, to taste.
- 3 sprigs thyme.

Directions:

1. Preheat the oven to 350º F.
2. Place ½ the sliced lemons on the bottom of a baking dish.
3. Place the salmon fillets over the lemons and cover with the remaining lemon slices and thyme.
4. Drizzle olive oil over the dish and cook for 20 minutes.
5. Season with salt and pepper.

Nutrition:

- **Calories:** 571 g.
- **Carbs:** 2 g.
- **Fats:** 44 g.
- **Protein:** 42 g.

59. Japanese Fish Bone Broth

Preparation Time: 5 minutes.

Cooking Time: 4 hours.

Servings: 6–8

Ingredients:

- 1 fish head and carcass.
- 4 slices ginger.
- 1 tbsp. lemon juice.
- ½ leek, sliced.
- Sea salt, to taste.
- Water.

Directions:

1. Place the fish head and carcass into a large pot with cold water.
2. Bring to a boil and pour out the water.
3. Refill the pot with fresh water and add in the leek, sea salt, ginger, and lemon juice.
4. Simmer, covered, about 4 hours.

Nutrition:

- **Calories:** 40 g.
- **Fats:** 2 g.
- **Protein:** 5 g.

60. Baked Garlic Ghee Chicken Breast

Preparation Time: 5 minutes.

Cooking Time: 30 minutes.

Servings: 1

Ingredients:

- 1 chicken breast
- 1 tsp. garlic powder
- 1 tbsp. ghee
- 2 garlic cloves, chopped
- 1 tsp. sea salt
- 1 tsp. chives, diced

Directions:

1. Preheat oven to 350º F.
2. Place the chicken breast on a piece of foil.
3. Season with sea salt, garlic powder, chopped fresh garlic.
4. Top with the ghee and rub everything into the chicken breast.
5. Wrap the chicken breast in the foil and place it on a baking tray.
6. Bake for 30 minutes, or until chicken breast is cooked through, with a meat thermometer reading above 165º F.
7. Serve with more salt and ghee to taste. Cut the chicken breast into slices and sprinkle the diced chives on top.

Nutrition:

- **Calories:** 264 g.
- **Carbs:** 6.1 g.
- **Fats:** 15.5 g.
- **Protein:** 23.7 g.

61. Crispy Oven Roasted Salmon

Preparation Time: 5 minutes.

Cooking Time: 20 minutes.

Servings: 3

Ingredients:

- 1 lb. salmon fillet.
- ¼ tsp. sea salt.
- 2 tbsps. coconut oil.
- ½ tsp. mixed herbs (oregano, thyme, marjoram).

Directions:

1. Preheat the oven to 425º F.
2. Line a baking sheet with parchment paper and grease with 1 tbsp. of coconut oil.
3. Place the salmon fillet on the lined baking sheet skin-side down.
4. Season with salt and herbs.
5. Place 1 tbsp. of coconut oil on top of the salmon.
6. Cook for 20 minutes or until your desired level of crispiness is reached.
7. Serve immediately.

Tip: You can store the dish in a glass container in the fridge for up to 2 days.

Nutrition:

- **Calories:** 400 g.
- **Carbs:** 0.2 g.
- **Fats:** 28.7 g.
- **Protein:** 35.8 g.

62. The Best Garlic Cilantro Salmon

Preparation Time: 10 minutes.

Cooking Time: 15 minutes.

Servings: 4

Ingredients:

- 1 lb. salmon filet.
- 1 tbsp. butter.
- 1 lemon.
- ¼ cup fresh cilantro leaves, chopped.
- 4 garlic cloves, minced.
- ½ tsp. kosher salt.
- ½ tsp. black pepper, freshly ground.

Directions:

1. Preheat the oven to 400º F.
2. On a foil-lined baking sheet, place the salmon fillet skin-side down.
3. Squeeze the lemon over the salmon.
4. Season the salmon with cilantro and garlic, pepper, and salt.
5. Slice the butter thinly and place pieces evenly over the salmon.
6. Bake for about 7 minutes, depending on thickness.
7. Turn the oven to "broil" and cook 5–7 minutes, or until the top is crispy.
8. Remove the salmon from the oven and serve immediately.

Nutrition:

- **Calories:** 140 g.
- **Carbs:** 3.5 g.
- **Fats:** 4 g.
- **Protein:** 24.9 g.

63. Pinchos de Pollo Marinated Grilled Chicken Kebabs

Preparation Time: 10 minutes (+2 hours).

Cooking Time: 10 minutes.

Servings: 4

Ingredients:

- 1 ½ lb. boneless, skinless chicken breast.
- 1 tbsp. minced garlic.
- ½ tsp. Himalayan salt, fine.
- ½ tsp. freshly ground black pepper.
- 1 tsp. dried oregano.
- 1 tbsp. extra-virgin olive oil.
- 1 lime juiced.
- 7–9 skewers.

Directions:

1. Have ready 7–9 soaked skewers.
2. In a bowl, combine the salt, garlic, pepper, lime juice, oregano, and oil.
3. Cut the chicken breast into 1-inch chunks and place it in a container with a lid.
4. Pour the marinade over the chicken and stir. Cover and refrigerate at least for 2 hours or overnight.
5. Preheat a grill to 325–375º F.
6. Remove the chicken from the refrigerator and thread it onto the skewers, leaving a very small space between each piece and spreading each piece as flat as possible.
7. Once the grill is hot, grill the kebabs over direct medium heat, about 8–10 minutes total, keeping the lid closed until the chicken is no longer pink in the center and is firm to the touch, turning once or twice during cooking. Take care not to overcook.
8. Remove from the grill and serve immediately!

Nutrition:

- **Calories:** 290 g.
- **Carbs:** 3 g.
- **Fats:** 10 g.
- **Protein:** 9 g.

64. Camembert Mushrooms

Preparation Time: 8 minutes.

Cooking Time: 5 minutes.

Servings: 3

Ingredients:

- 2 tbsps. butter.
- 4 oz. Camembert cheese, diced.
- 2 tsp. garlic, minced.
- 1 lb. button mushrooms, halved.
- Black pepper to taste.

Directions:

1. Place a skillet over medium-high heat. Add the butter and let it melt. Once the butter has melted, add the garlic and sauté until translucent; it should take 3 minutes. Add the mushrooms and cheese and cook for 10 minutes. Season with pepper and serve. Enjoy!

Nutrition:

- **Calories:** 161g.
- **Fats:** 13 g.
- **Carbs:** 3 g.
- **Protein:** 9 g.

65. Mediterranean Stuffed Chicken

Preparation Time: 35 minutes.

Cooking Time: 25 minutes.

Servings: 2

Ingredients:

- 2 skinless and boneless chicken breast halves.
- ¼ cup feta cheese, crumbled.
- 2 tbsps. red sweet peppers, finely chopped, roasted.
- 15 oz. bell peppers, roasted.
- 2 tbsps. green onion, thinly sliced.
- 2 tbsps. snipped fresh oregano.
- ½ tsp. oregano, crushed, dried.
- ½ tsp. black pepper, ground.

Directions:

1. In each chicken breast, cut a pocket, usually in the thickest part, then put the chicken breast aside.
2. Take a bowl and mix it in with the feta cheese, roasted peppers, oregano, and green onion. Stuff the pockets of the chicken breasts with the mixture you now have.
3. Place the chicken breast into a frying pan and let them cook over medium heat. When cooked, the chicken breast will turn white (from pink), and the temperature of the thickest part should be around 170º F. As an alternative, you can use a grill, but the instructions are still the same.
4. After around 15 minutes over medium heat, you will need to flip over the chicken breasts (halfway through) and let them grill for 10 more minutes. Put the chicken aside and let it cool. We recommend veggies as a side dish, but it's really your call if you feel like using rice, or potatoes.

Nutrition:

- **Calories:** 186 g.
- **Fats:** 8.6 g.
- **Saturated fats:** 2.6 g.
- **Cholesterol:** 57.1 mg.
- **Sodium:** 334.7 mg.
- **Carbs:** 1.5 g.
- **Sugar:** 0.9 g.
- **Fiber:** 0.1 g.
- **Protein:** 23.4 g.

66. Vegan Tuna Salad

Preparation Time: 5 minutes.

Cooking Time: 55 minutes.

Servings: 6

Ingredients:

- 2 cans of chickpeas.
- 1 tbsp. prepared yellow mustard.
- 2 tbsps. vegan mayonnaise.
- 1 tbsp. jarred capers.
- 2 tbsps. pickle relish.
- ½ cup chopped celery.

Directions:

1. In a medium bowl, combine chickpeas, mustard, vegan mayo, and capers. Pulse in a food processor or mash with a potato masher until the mixture is partially smooth with some chunks.
2. Add the remaining ingredients to the chickpea mixture and mix until combined.
3. Serve immediately or refrigerate until ready to serve.

Nutrition:

- **Calories:** 170 g.
- **Fat:** 18 g.
- **Protein:** 15 g.
- **Carbs:** 1.8 g.

67. Veggie Wrap With Apples and Spicy Hummus

Preparation Time: 5 minutes.

Cooking Time: 40 minutes.

Servings: 6

Ingredients:

- 1 tortilla of your choice: flour, corn, gluten-free, etc.
- 3–4 tbsps. your favorite spicy hummus (a plain hummus mixed with salsa is good, too!)
- A few leaves of your favorite leafy greens.
- ¼ apple sliced thin.
- ½ cup broccoli slaw (store-bought or homemade are both good).
- ½ tsp. lemon juice.
- 2 tsps. dairy-free, plain, unsweetened yogurt.
- Salt and pepper to taste.

Directions:

1. Mix broccoli slaw with lemon juice and yogurt. Add pepper and salt to taste and mix well.
2. Lay tortilla flat.
3. Spread hummus all over the tortilla.
4. Lay down leafy greens on hummus.
5. On one half, pile broccoli slaw over lettuce. Place apples on top of the slaw.
6. Starting with the half with slaw and apples, roll the tortilla tightly.
7. Cut in half if desired and enjoy!

Nutrition:

- **Calories:** 110 g.
- **Fat:** 8 g.
- **Protein:** 15 g.
- **Carbs:** 8 g.

68. Turmeric Rack of Lamb

Preparation Time: 15 minutes.

Cooking Time: 16 minutes.

Servings: 4

Ingredients:

- 13 oz. rack of lamb.
- 1 tbsp. ground turmeric.
- ½ tsp. chili flakes.
- 3 tbsps. olive oil.
- 1 tbsp. balsamic vinegar.
- 1 tsp. salt.
- ½ tsp. peppercorns.
- ¾ cup of water.

Directions:

1. In the shallow bowl, mix up together ground turmeric, chili flakes, olive oil, balsamic vinegar, salt, and peppercorns.
2. Brush the rack of lamb with the oily mixture generously.
3. After this, preheat the grill to 380º F.
4. Place the rack of lamb in the grill and cook it for 8 minutes from each side.
5. The cooked rack of lamb should have a light crunchy crust.

Nutrition:

- **Calories:** 190 g.
- **Fat:** 28 g.
- **Protein:** 15 g.
- **Carbs:** 8 g.

69. Sausage Casserole

Preparation Time: 10 minutes.

Cooking Time: 35 minutes.

Servings: 6

Ingredients:

- 2 jalapeno peppers, sliced.
- 5 oz. cheddar cheese, shredded.
- 9 oz. sausages, chopped.
- 1 tbsp. olive oil.
- ½ cup spinach, chopped.
- ½ cup heavy cream.
- ½ tsp. salt.

Directions:

1. Brush the casserole mold with olive oil from inside.
2. Then put the chopped sausages in the casserole mold in one layer.
3. Add chopped spinach and sprinkle it with salt.
4. After this, add sliced jalapeno pepper.
5. Then make the layer of shredded cheddar cheese.
6. Pour the heavy cream over the cheese.
7. Preheat the oven to 355º F.
8. Transfer the casserole to the oven and cook it for 35 minutes.
9. Use the kitchen torch to make the crunchy cheese crust of the casserole.

Nutrition:

- **Calories:** 150 g.
- **Fat:** 18 g.
- **Protein:** 15 g.
- **Carbs:** 1.8 g.

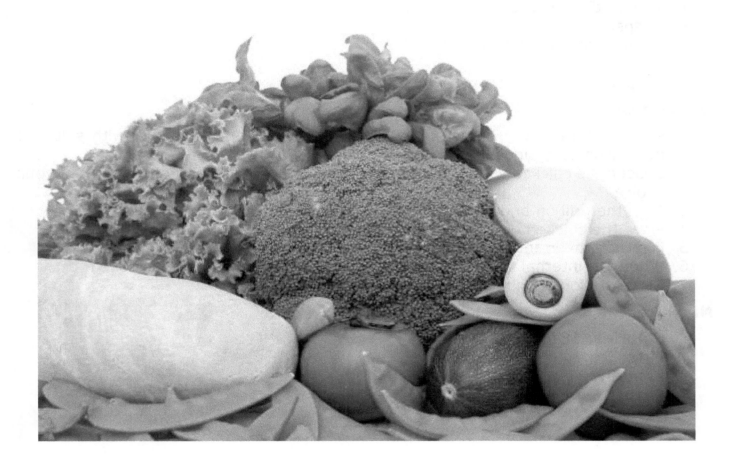

Dinner

70. Garlic Herb Grilled Chicken Breast

Preparation Time: 7 minutes.

Cooking Time: 20 minutes.

Servings: 4

Ingredients:

- 1 ¼ lb. chicken breasts, skinless and boneless.
- 2 tsps. olive oil.
- 1 tbsp. garlic & herb seasoning blend.
- Salt.
- Pepper.

Directions:

1. Pat dry the chicken breasts, coat it with olive oil, and season it with salt and pepper on both sides.
2. Season the chicken with garlic and herb seasoning or any other seasoning of your choice.
3. Turn the grill on and oil the grate.
4. Place the chicken on the hot grate and let it grill till the sides turn white.
5. Flip them over and let them cook again.
6. When the internal temperature is about 160º F, it is most likely cooked.
7. Set aside for 15 minutes. Chop into pieces.

Nutrition:

- **Calories:** 187 g.
- **Fats:** 6 g.
- **Protein:** 32 g.
- **Carbs:** 5 g.

71. Cajun Shrimp

Preparation Time: 10 minutes.

Cooking Time: 5 minutes.

Servings: 2

Ingredients:

- 16 tiger shrimp.
- 2 tbsps. corn starch.
- 1 tsp. cayenne pepper.
- 1 tsp. old bay seasoning.
- 1 tsp. olive oil.
- Salt.
- Pepper.

Directions:

1. Rinse the shrimp. Pat dry.
2. In a bowl, combine corn starch, cayenne pepper, old bay seasoning, salt, pepper. Stir.
3. In a bowl, add the shrimp. Drizzle olive oil over shrimp to lightly coat.
4. Dip the shrimp in seasoning, shake off any excess.
5. Preheat fryer to 375º F. Lightly spray cook basket with non-stick keto cooking spray.
6. Transfer to the fryer. Cook 5 minutes; shake after 2 minutes, until cooked thoroughly.
7. Serve on a platter.

Nutrition:

- **Calories:** 127 g.
- **Fat:** 10 g.
- **Carbs:** 3 g.
- **Protein:** 7 g.

72. Sesame-Crusted Mahi-Mahi

Preparation Time: 5 minutes.

Cooking Time: 13 minutes.

Servings: 4

Ingredients:

- 2 tbsps. Dijon mustard.
- 1 tbsp. sour cream, low-fat.
- ½ cup sesame seeds.
- 2 tbsps. olive oil.
- 1 lemon, wedged.
- 4 (4 oz. each) mahi-mahi or sole filets.

Directions:

1. Rinse filets and pat dry. In a bowl, mix sour cream and mustard. Spread this mixture on all sides of the fish. Roll in sesame seeds to coat.
2. Heat olive oil in a large skillet over medium heat. Pan-fry fish, turning once, for 5–8 minutes or until fish flakes when tested with fork and sesame seeds are toasted. Serve immediately with lemon wedges.

Nutrition:

- **Calories:** 282 g.
- **Fat:** 17 g.
- **Protein:** 18 g.
- **Carbs:** 5 g.

73. Country Chicken

Preparation Time: 10 minutes.

Cooking Time: 15 minutes.

Servings: 2

Ingredients:

- ¾ lbs. chicken tenders, fresh, boneless skinless.
- ½ cup almond meal.
- ½ cup almond flour.
- 1 tsp. rosemary, dried.
- Salt.
- Pepper.
- 2 eggs, beaten.

Directions:

1. Rinse the chicken tenders, pat dry.
2. In a medium bowl, pour in almond flour.
3. In a medium bowl, beat the eggs.
4. In a separate bowl, pour in an almond meal. Season with rosemary, salt, pepper.
5. Take the chicken pieces and toast in flour, then egg, then almond meal. Set on a tray.
6. Place the tray in the freezer for 5 minutes.
7. Preheat fryer to 350° F. Lightly spray cook basket with non-stick cooking spray.
8. Cook tenders for 10 minutes. After the timer runs out, set the temperature to 390° F, cook for 5 more minutes until golden brown.
9. Serve on a platter. Side with preferred dipping sauce.

Nutrition:

- **Calories:** 480 g.
- **Fat:** 36 g.
- **Carbs:** 13 g.
- **Protein:** 26 g.

74. Mahi-Mahi Tacos With Avocado and Fresh Cabbage

Preparation Time: 5 minutes.

Cooking Time: 15 minutes.

Servings: 4

Ingredients:

- 1 lb. mahi-mahi.
- Salt.
- Pepper.
- 1 tsp. olive oil.
- 1 avocado.
- 4 corn tortillas.
- 2 cups cabbage, shredded.
- 2 quartered limes.

Directions:

1. Season fish with salt and pepper.
2. Set a pan over medium-high heat. Add in oil and heat. Once the oil is hot, sauté fish for about 3–4 minutes on each side. Slice or flake fish into 1-oz. pieces.
3. Slice avocado in half. Remove seed and, using a spoon, remove the flesh from the skin. Slice the avocado halves into ½ thick slices.
4. In a small pan, warm corn tortillas; cook for about 1 minute on each side.
5. Place one-fourth of Mahi-mahi of each tortilla, top with avocado and cabbage. Serve with lime wedges.

Nutrition:

- **Calories:** 251 g.
- **Fat:** 9 g.
- **Protein:** 25 g.
- **Carbs:** 21 g.

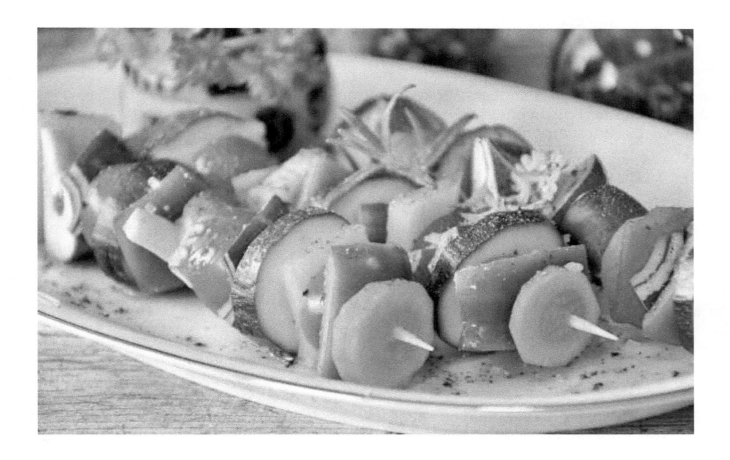

75. Butternut Squash Risotto

Preparation Time: 10 minutes.

Cooking Time: 15 minutes.

Servings: 4

Ingredients:

- 3 tbsps. butter.
- 2 tbsps. minced sage.
- ¼ tsp. black pepper, ground.
- 1 tsp. minced rosemary.
- 1 tsp. salt.
- ½ cup dry sherry.
- 4 cups riced cauliflower.
- ½ cup butternut squash, cooked and mashed.
- ½ cup parmesan cheese, grated.
- ½ cup mascarpone cheese.
- $1/8$ tsp. grated nutmeg.
- 1 tsp. minced garlic.

Directions:

1. Melt your butter inside of a large frying pan turned to a medium level of heat.
2. Add your rosemary, your sage, and the garlic. Cook this for about 1 minute or until this mixture begins to become fragrant.
3. Add in the cauliflower rice, pepper and salt, and the mashed squash. Cook this for 3 minutes. You will know it is ready for the next step when cauliflower is starting to soften up for you.
4. Add in your sherry and cook this for an additional 6 minutes, or until the majority of the liquid is absorbed into the rice, or when the cauliflower is much softer.
5. Stir in the mascarpone cheese, the parmesan cheese, as well as the nutmeg (grated).
6. Cook all of this on a medium heat level, being sure to stir it occasionally and do this until the cheese has melted and the risotto has gotten creamy. This will take around 4–5 minutes.
7. Taste the risotto and add more pepper and salt to season if you wish.
8. Remove your pan from the burner and garnish your risotto with more of the herbs as well as some grated parmesan.
9. Serve and enjoy

Nutrition: 5

- **Calories:** 337 g.
- **Fats:** 25 g.
- **Carbs:** 9 g.
- **Protein:** 8 g.

76. Cheesy Broccoli Soup

Preparation Time: 5 minutes.

Cooking Time: 30 minutes.

Servings: 6

Ingredients:

- 2 lbs. broccoli, chopped.
- Salt to taste.
- 5 cups vegetable broth.
- ¼ cup shredded cheddar cheese.
- 1 tbsp. olive oil.
- ¼ cup lemon juice.
- 2 garlic cloves, mince.
- 1 white onion, chopped.
- Pepper to taste.

Directions:

1. Heat the olive oil in a pan with medium heat.
2. Fry the onion for 1 minute and then add the garlic. Fry until the garlic becomes golden in color.
3. Toss in the broccoli and stir for 3 minutes.
4. Pour in the vegetable broth.
5. Add salt, pepper and mix well.
6. Cook for 20 minutes or until your broccoli is perfectly cooked through.
7. Take off the heat and let it cool down a bit.
8. Add to a blender, and blend it until your soup is perfectly smooth.
9. Transfer the soup into the pot again and heat it over medium heat.
10. Add lemon juice, cheddar cheese, and check if it needs more seasoning.
11. Serve hot with more cheese on top.

Nutrition:

- **Calories:** 97 g.
- **Fats:** 3.6 g.
- **Carbs:** 13.4 g.
- **Proteins:** 5 g.

77. Beef Cabbage Stew

Preparation Time: 30 minutes.

Cooking Time: 2 hours.

Servings: 8

Ingredients:

- 2 lbs. beef stew meat.
- 1 cube beef bouillon.
- 8-oz. tomato sauce.
- ¼ cup chopped celery.
- 2 bay leaves.
- 8-oz. plum tomatoes, chopped.
- 1 $1/3$ cups hot chicken broth.
- Salt and pepper to taste.
- 1 cabbage.
- 1 tsp. Greek seasoning.
- 4 onions, chopped.

Directions:

1. Cut off the stem of the cabbage. Separate the leaves carefully. Wash well and rinse off. Set aside for now.
2. Fry the beef in a large pan over medium-low heat for about 8–10 minutes or until you get a brown color.
3. Into the pan, pour in $1/3$ of the chicken broth.
4. Add the beef bouillon, and mix well.
5. Add the black pepper, salt and mix again.
6. Add the lid and cook on medium-low heat for about 1 hour.
7. Take off the heat and transfer the mix into a bowl.
8. Spread the cabbage leaves on a flat surface.
9. Fill the middle using the beef mixture. Use a generous portion of filling, it will give your stew a better taste.
10. Wrap the cabbage leaves tightly. Use a kitchen thread to tie it. Finish it with the remaining leaves and filling.
11. In a pot heat the oil over fry the onion for 1 minute.
12. Add the remaining chicken broth.
13. Add in the celery and tomato sauce and cook for another 10 minutes.
14. Add the Greek seasonings, and mix well. Bring to boil and then carefully add the wrapped cabbage.
15. Cover and cook for another 10 minutes.
16. Serve hot.

Nutrition:

- **Calories:** 372 g.
- **Fats:** 22.7 g.
- **Carbs:** 9 g.
- **Protein:** 31.8 g.

78. Fried Whole Tilapia

Preparation Time: 10 minutes.

Cooking Time: 25 minutes.

Servings: 2

Ingredients:

- 10-oz. tilapia.
- 2 tbsps. oil.
- 5 garlic cloves, mince.
- 4 large onions, chopped.
- 2 tbsps. red chili powder.
- 1 tsp. turmeric powder.
- 1 tsp. cumin powder.
- 1 tsp. coriander powder.
- Salt to taste.
- Black pepper to taste.
- 2 tbsps. soy sauce.
- 2 tbsps. fish sauce.

Directions:

1. Take the tilapia fish and clean it well without taking off the skin. You need to fry it whole, so you have to be careful about cleaning the gut inside.
2. Cut few slits on the skin so the seasoning gets inside well.
3. Marinate the fish with fish sauce, soy sauce, red chili powder, cumin powder, turmeric powder, coriander powder, salt, and pepper.
4. Coat half of the onions in the same mixture too.
5. Let them marinate for 1 hour.
6. In a skillet heat the oil. Fry the fish for 8 minutes on each side.
7. Transfer the fish to a serving plate.
8. Fry the marinated onions until they become crispy.
9. Add the remaining raw onions on top and serve hot.

Nutrition:

- **Calories:** 368 g.
- **Fats:** 30.1 g.
- **Carbs:** 9.2 g.
- **Proteins:** 16.6 g.

79. African Chicken Curry

Preparation Time: 10 minutes.

Cooking Time: 30 minutes.

Servings: 4

Ingredients:

- 1 lb. whole chicken.
- ½ onion.
- ½ cup coconut milk.
- ½ bay leaf.
- 1 ½ tsps. olive oil.
- ½ cup peeled tomatoes.
- 1 tsp. curry powder.
- $\frac{1}{8}$ tsp. salt.
- ½ lemon, juiced.
- 1 clove garlic.

Directions:

1. Keep the skin of the chicken.
2. Cut your chicken into 8 pieces. It looks good when you keep the size not too small or not too big.
3. Discard the skin of the onion and garlic and mince the garlic and dice the onion.
4. Cut the tomato wedges.
5. Now in a pot add the olive oil and heat over medium heat.
6. Add the garlic and fry until it becomes brown.
7. Add the diced onion and caramelize it.
8. Add the bay leaf, and chicken pieces.
9. Fry the chicken pieces until they are golden.
10. Add the curry powder, coconut milk, and salt.
11. Cover and cook for 10 minutes on high heat.
12. Lower the heat to medium-low and add the lemon juice.
13. Add the tomato wedges and coconut milk.
14. Cook for another 10 minutes.
15. Serve hot with rice or tortilla.

Nutrition:

- **Calories:** 354 g.
- **Fats:** 10 g.
- **Proteins:** 18 g.
- **Carbs:** 17 g.

80. Yummy Garlic Chicken Livers

Preparation Time: 10 minutes.

Cooking Time: 30 minutes.

Servings: 2

Ingredients:

- ½ lb. chicken liver.
- 2 tsp. lime juice.
- 6 garlic cloves, mince.
- ½ tsp. salt.
- 1 tbsp. ginger-garlic paste.
- 1 cup diced onion.
- 1 tbsp. red chili powder.
- 1 tsp. cumin.
- 1 tsp. coriander powder.
- Black pepper to taste.
- 1 cardamom.
- 2 tomatoes.
- 1 cinnamon stick.
- 1 bay leaf.
- 4 tbsp. olive oil.

Directions:

1. In a large pan, heat your oil over high heat.
2. Add the garlic and fry them golden brown.
3. Add onion and fry until they become caramelized.
4. Turn the heat to medium and add the bay leaf, cinnamon stick, cardamom, and toss for 30 seconds.
5. Add the ginger-garlic paste and 1 tbsp. water. Adding water prevents burning.
6. Add the coriander powder, black pepper, salt, cumin, and red chili powder.
7. Cover and cook for 3 minutes on low heat.
8. Add the livers and cook on medium heat for 15 minutes.
9. Add the tomatoes and cook for another 5 minutes.
10. Check the seasoning, add more salt if needed.
11. Serve hot with the tortilla.

Nutrition:

- **Calories:** 174 g.
- **Fats:** 9 g.
- **Protein:** 18 g.
- **Carbs:** 2.4 g.

81. Healthy Chickpea Burger

Preparation Time: 15 minutes.

Cooking Time: 10 minutes.

Servings: 2

Ingredients:

- 1 cup chickpeas, boiled.
- 1 tbsp. tomato puree.
- 1 tsp. soy sauce.
- A pinch of paprika.
- A pinch of white pepper.
- 1 onion, diced.
- Salt to taste.
- 2 lettuce leaves.
- ½ cup bell pepper, sliced.
- 1 tsp. olive oil.
- 1 avocado, sliced.
- 2 burger buns to serve.

Directions:

1. Mash the chickpeas and combine with bell pepper, salt, pepper, paprika, soy sauce, and tomato puree.
2. Use your hands to make patties.
3. Fry the patties golden brown with oil.
4. Assemble the burgers with lettuce, onion, avocado, and enjoy.

Nutrition:

- **Calories:** 254 g.
- **Fat:** 12 g.
- **Protein:** 9 g.
- **Carbs:** 7.8 g.

82. Quinoa Protein Bars

Preparation Time: 15 minutes.

Cooking Time: 40 minutes.

Servings: 16

Ingredients:

- ½ cup almonds, chopped.
- ½ cup chocolate chips.
- ½ cup coconut oil, melted.
- ½ cup flaxseed, ground.
- ½ cup honey.
- ½ tsp. salt.
- 1 cup quinoa, dry.
- 2 ¼ cups quick oats.
- 3 large egg whites.

Directions:

1. Preheat oven to 325º F
2. On the bottom of a clean, dry baking sheet evenly spread oats, quinoa, and almonds.
3. Bake for about 15 minutes or until lightly brown. You may want to stir the items in the cookie sheet every few minutes to ensure nothing burns.
4. Remove grains and nuts from the oven and allow to cool completely, but don't turn off the oven.
5. Whisk the egg whites in a bowl and beat the coconut oil and honey into them.
6. Combine flaxseed, chocolate chips, and salt into the cooled grains and nuts, and then pour that mixture into the mixing bowl, coating everything completely.
7. Line your baking sheet with parchment paper and spread the mixture evenly onto it, pressing it into one even layer. You may want to shape the sides of the mass, depending on whether or not it reaches the edges of your baking sheet without thinning out too much.
8. Bake for 30 minutes, then remove from the oven.
9. Let cool for one hour before slicing into evenly-shaped bars, then cool completely.
10.   Enjoy!

Nutrition:

- **Calories:** 269 g.
- **Carbs:** 30 g.
- **Fats:** 15 g.
- **Protein:** 6 g.

83. Mediterranean Lamb

Preparation Time: 10 minutes.

Cooking Time: 35 minutes.

Servings: 4

Ingredients:

- 2 ½ lbs. lamb shoulder, cut into chunks.
- 1 bay leaf.
- 1 cup vegetable stock.
- 10 oz. prunes, soaked.
- 1 tsp. garlic, minced.
- 2 tbsp. honey.
- 2 onions, sliced.
- 1 tsp. ground cumin.
- 1 tsp. ground ginger.
- 1 tsp. ground turmeric.
- ¼ tsp. cinnamon.
- 3 oz. almonds sliced.
- Pepper.
- Salt.

Directions:

1. Add all ingredients into the inner pot of the Instant Pot and stir well.
2. Seal pot with lid and cook on high for 35 minutes.
3. Once done, allow to release pressure naturally. Remove lid.
4. Serve and enjoy.

Nutrition:

- **Calories:** 870 g.
- **Fat:** 34 g.
- **Fiber:** 4 g.
- **Carbs:** 30 g.
- **Protein:** 86 g.

84. Coated Cauliflower Head

Preparation Time: 10 minutes.

Cooking Time: 40 minutes.

Servings: 6

Ingredients:

- 2-lb. cauliflower head.
- 3 tbsps. olive oil.
- 1 tbsp. butter softened.
- 1 tsp. ground coriander.
- 1 tsp. salt.
- 1 egg, whisked.
- 1 tsp. dried cilantro.
- 1 tsp. dried oregano.
- 1 tsp. Tahini paste.

Directions:

1. Trim cauliflower head if needed.
2. Preheat oven to 350º F.
3. In the mixing bowl, mix up together olive oil, softened butter, ground coriander, salt, whisked egg, dried cilantro, dried oregano, and tahini paste.
4. Then brush the cauliflower head with this mixture generously and transfer it to the tray.
5. Bake the cauliflower head for 40 minutes.
6. Brush it with the remaining oil mixture every 10 minutes.

Nutrition:

- **Calories:** 131 g.
- **Fat:** 10.3 g.
- **Fiber:** 4 g.
- **Carbs:** 8.4 g.
- **Protein:** 4.1 g.

85. Artichoke Petals Bites

Preparation Time: 10 minutes.

Cooking Time: 10 minutes.

Servings: 8

Ingredients:

- 8 oz. artichoke petals, boiled, drained, without salt.
- ½ cup almond flour.
- 4 oz. Parmesan, grated.
- 2 tbsps. almond butter, melted.

Directions:

1. In the mixing bowl, mix up together almond flour and grated Parmesan.
2. Preheat the oven to 355º F.
3. Dip the artichoke petals in the almond butter and then coat in the almond flour mixture.
4. Place them in the tray.
5. Transfer the tray to the preheated oven and cook the petals for 10 minutes.
6. Chill the cooked petal bites a little before serving.

Nutrition:

- **Calories:** 140 g.
- **Fat:** 6.4 g.
- **Fiber:** 7.6 g.
- **Carbs:** 14.6 g.
- **Protein:** 10 g.

86. Stuffed Beef Loin in Sticky Sauce

Preparation Time: 15 minutes.

Cooking Time: 6 minutes.

Servings: 4

Ingredients:

- 1 tbsp. Erythritol.
- 1 tbsp. lemon juice.
- ½ tsp. tomato sauce.
- ¼ tsp. dried rosemary.
- 9 oz. beef loin.
- 3 oz. celery root, grated.
- 3 oz. bacon, sliced.
- 1 tbsp. walnuts, chopped.
- ¾ tsps. garlic, diced.
- 2 tsps. butter.
- 1 tbsp. olive oil.
- 1 tsp. salt.
- ½ cup of water.

Directions:

1. Cut the beef loin into the layer and spread it with the dried rosemary, butter, and salt.
2. Then place over the beef loin: grated celery root, sliced bacon, walnuts, and diced garlic.
3. Roll the beef loin and brush it with olive oil.
4. Secure the meat with the help of the toothpicks.
5. Place it in the tray and add a ½ cup of water.
6. Cook the meat in the preheated to 365º F oven for 40 minutes.
7. Meanwhile, make the sticky sauce: mix up together Erythritol, lemon juice, 4 tbsps. of water, and butter.
8. Preheat the mixture until it starts to boil.
9. Then add tomato sauce and whisk it well.
10. Bring the sauce to boil and remove from the heat.
11. When the beef loin is cooked, remove it from the oven and brush it with the cooked sticky sauce very generously.
12. Slice the beef roll and sprinkle with the remaining sauce.

Nutrition:

- **Calories:** 248 g.
- **Fat:** 17.5 g.
- **Fiber:** 0.5 g.
- **Carbs:** 2.2 g.
- **Protein:** 20.7 g.

87. Olive Feta Beef

Preparation Time: 10 minutes.

Cooking Time: 6 hours.

Servings: 8

Ingredients:

- 2 lbs. beef stew meat, cut into half-inch pieces.
- 1 cup olives, pitted, and cut in half.
- 30 oz. can tomatoes, diced.
- ½ cup feta cheese, crumbled.
- ¼ tsp. pepper.
- ½ tsp. salt.

Directions:

1. Add all ingredients into the crockpot and stir well.
2. Cover and cook on high for 6 hours.
3. Season with pepper and salt.
4. Stir well and serve.

Nutrition:

- **Calories:** 370 g.
- **Fat:** 12 g.
- **Fiber:** 1 g.
- **Carbs:** 10 g.
- **Protein:** 50 g.

88. Italian Beef Casserole

Preparation Time: 10 minutes.

Cooking Time: 1 hour 30 minutes.

Servings: 6

Ingredients:

- 1 lb. lean stew beef, cut into chunks.
- 3 tsps. paprika.
- 4 oz. black olives, sliced.
- 7 oz. can tomatoes, chopped.
- 1 tbsp. tomato puree.
- ¼ tsp. garlic powder.
- 2 tsps. herb de Provence.
- 2 cups beef stock.
- 2 tbsps. olive oil.

Directions:

1. Preheat the oven to 350º F.
2. Heat oil in a pan over medium heat.
3. Add meat to the pan and cook until brown.
4. Add stock, olives, tomatoes, tomato puree, garlic powder, herb de Provence, and paprika. Stir well and bring to boil.
5. Transfer the meat mixture to the casserole dish.
6. Cover and cook in preheated oven for 1 ½ hour.
7. Serve and enjoy.

Nutrition:

- **Calories:** 100 g.
- **Fat:** 7 g.
- **Fiber:** 2 g.
- **Carbs:** 8 g.
- **Protein:** 6 g.

89. Chicken With Kale and Chili Salsa

Preparation Time: 5 minutes.

Cooking Time: 45 minutes.

Servings: 1

Ingredients:

- 3 oz. buckwheat.
- 1 tsp. chopped fresh ginger.
- Juice of ½ lemon, divided.
- 2 tsps. ground turmeric.
- 3 oz. kale, chopped.
- 1.3 oz. red onion, sliced.
- 4 oz. skinless, boneless chicken breast.
- 1 tbsp. extra-virgin olive oil.
- 1 tomato.
- 1 handful parsley.
- 1 bird's eye chili, chopped.

Directions:

2. Start with the salsa: Remove the eye out of the tomato and finely chop it, making sure to keep as much of the liquid as you can. Mix it with chili, parsley, and lemon juice. You could add everything to a blender for different results.
3. Heat your oven to 220º F. Marinate the chicken with a little oil, 1 tsp. of turmeric, and lemon juice. Let it rest for 5–10 minutes.
4. Heat a pan over medium heat until it is hot then add marinated chicken and allow it to cook for a minute on both sides (until it is pale gold). Transfer the chicken to the oven if the pan is not ovenproof, place it in a baking tray and bake for 8–10 minutes or until it is cooked through. Take the chicken out of the oven, cover with foil, and let it rest for 5 minutes before you serve.
5. Meanwhile, in a steamer, steam the kale for about 5 minutes.
6. In a little oil, fry the ginger and red onions until they are soft but not colored, and then add in the cooked kale and fry it for a minute.
7. Cook the buckwheat in accordance with the packet directions with the remaining turmeric. Serve alongside the vegetables, salsa, and chicken.

Nutrition:

- **Calories:** 134.8 g.
- **Fat:** 30 g.
- **Protein:** 56 g.
- **Carbs:** 45 g.
- **Cholesterol:** 230 mg.
- **Sugar:** 0 g.

90. Buckwheat Tuna Casserole

Preparation Time: 10 minutes.

Cooking Time: 35 minutes.

Servings: 2

Ingredients:

- 2 tbsps. butter.
- 10-oz. package buckwheat ramen noodles.
- 2 cups boiling water.
- $\frac{1}{3}$ cup dry red wine.
- 3 cups milk.
- 2 tbsps. dried parsley.
- 2 tsps. turmeric.
- ½ tsp. curry powder.
- 2 tbsps. all-purpose flour.
- 2 cups celery, chopped.
- 1 cup frozen peas.
- 2 cans of tuna, drained.

Directions:

1. Dot butter into your crockpot and grease the pot.
2. Place buckwheat ramen noodles in a large bowl and pour boiling water to cover. Let sit for 5–8 minutes, or until noodles separate when prodded with a fork.
3. In a separate bowl, whisk together red wine, milk, parsley, turmeric, and flour.
4. Fold in celery, peas, and tuna.
5. Drain the ramen and place it into the crockpot, pouring the tuna mixture over top. Mix to combine.
6. Cover and cook on Low 7–9 hours, stirring occasionally.

Nutrition:

- **Calories:** 411 g.
- **Fat:** 30 g.
- **Protein:** 56 g.
- **Carbs:** 75 g.
- **Cholesterol:** 230 mg.
- **Sugar:** 0 g.

91. Cheesy Crockpot Chicken and Vegetables

Preparation Time: 10 minutes.

Cooking Time: 45 minutes.

Servings: 2

Ingredients:

- $1/3$ cup ham, diced.
- 3 carrots, chopped.
- 3 stalks celery, chopped.
- 1 small yellow onion, diced.
- 2 cups mushrooms, sliced.
- 1 cup green beans, chopped.
- ¼ cup water.
- 4 boneless, skinless chicken breasts, cubed.
- 1 cup chicken broth.
- 1 cup milk.
- 1 tbsp. parsley, chopped.
- ¾ tsps. poultry seasoning.
- 1 tbsp. all-purpose flour.
- 1 cup cheddar cheese, shredded.
- ¼ cup Parmesan, shredded.

Directions:

1. In a large bowl, combine ham, carrots, celery, onion, mushrooms, and green beans. Mix and transfer to your crockpot.
2. Layer the chicken on top, without mixing.
3. In the bowl, now empty, whisk broth, milk, parsley, poultry seasoning, and flour together until well combined.
4. Fold in the cheddar and Parmesan.
5. Pour the mixture over the chicken. DO NOT STIR.
6. Cover and cook on high 3–4 hours, or low 6–8 hours.

Nutrition:

- **Calories:** 417 g.
- **Fat:** 10 g.
- **Protein:** 56 g.
- **Carbs:** 45 g.
- **Cholesterol:** 230 mg.
- **Sugar:** 0 g.

92. Artichoke, Chicken, and Capers

Preparation Time: 10 minutes.

Cooking Time: 55 minutes.

Servings: 2

Ingredients:

- 6 boneless, skinless chicken breasts.
- 2 cups mushrooms, sliced.
- 1 (14 ½ oz.) can diced tomatoes.
- 1 (8 or 9 oz.) package frozen artichokes.
- 1 cup chicken broth.
- ¼ cup dry white wine.
- 1 medium yellow onion, diced.
- ½ cup Kalamata olives, sliced.
- ¼ cup capers, drained.
- 3 tbsps. chia seeds.
- 3 tsps. curry powder.
- 1 tsp. turmeric.
- ¾ tsps. dried lovage.
- Salt and pepper to taste.
- 3 cups hot cooked buckwheat.

Directions:

1. Rinse chicken & set aside.
2. In a large bowl, combine mushrooms, tomatoes (with juice), frozen artichoke hearts, chicken broth, white wine, onion, olives, and capers.
3. Stir in chia seeds, curry powder, turmeric, lovage, salt, and pepper.
4. Pour half the mixture into your crockpot, add the chicken, and pour the remainder of the sauce over top.
5. Cover and cook on low for 7–8 hours or on High for 3 ½ to 4 hours.
6. Serve with hot cooked buckwheat.

Nutrition:

- **Calories:** 473 g.
- **Protein:** 20 g.
- **Fat:** 3 g.
- **Carbs:** 15 g.

93. Chicken Merlot With Mushrooms

Preparation Time: 10 minutes.

Cooking Time: 40 minutes.

Servings: 2

Ingredients:

- 6 boneless, skinless chicken breasts, cubed.
- 3 cups mushrooms, sliced.
- 1 large red onion, chopped.
- 2 cloves garlic, minced.
- ¾ cup chicken broth.
- 1 (6 oz.) can tomato paste.
- ¼ cup Merlot.
- 3 tbsps. chia seeds.
- 2 tbsps. basil, chopped finely.
- 2 tsps. sugar.
- Salt and pepper to taste.
- 1 (10 oz.) package buckwheat ramen noodles, cooked.
- 2 tbsps. Parmesan, shaved.

Directions:

1. Rinse chicken; set aside.
2. Add mushrooms, onion, and garlic to the crockpot and mix.
3. Place chicken cubes on top of the vegetables and do not mix.
4. In a large bowl, combine broth, tomato paste, wine, chia seeds, basil, sugar, salt, and pepper. Pour over the chicken.
5. Cover and cook on low for 7–8 hours or on high for 3 ½–4 hours.
6. To serve, spoon chicken, mushroom mixture, and sauce over hot cooked buckwheat ramen noodles. Top with shaved Parmesan.

Nutrition:

- **Calories:** 213 g.
- **Fat:** 10 g.
- **Protein:** 56 g.
- **Carbs:** 45 g.
- **Cholesterol:** 230 mg.
- **Sugar:** 0 g.

94. Country Chicken Breasts

Preparation Time: 10 minutes.

Cooking Time: 45 minutes.

Servings: 2

Ingredients:

- 2 medium green apples, diced.
- 1 small red onion, finely diced.
- 1 small green bell pepper, chopped.
- 3 cloves garlic, minced.
- 2 tbsps. dried currants.
- 1 tbsp. curry powder.
- 1 tsp. turmeric.
- 1 tsp. ground ginger.
- ¼ tsp. chili pepper flakes.
- 1 can (14 ½ oz.) diced tomatoes.
- 6 skinless, boneless chicken breasts, halved.
- ½ cup chicken broth.
- 1 cup long-grain white rice.
- 1-lb. large raw shrimp, shelled and deveined.
- Salt and pepper to taste.
- Chopped parsley. $^{1}/_{3}$ cup slivered almonds.

Directions:

1. Rinse chicken, pat dry, and set aside.
2. In a large crockpot, combine apples, onion, bell pepper, garlic, currants, curry powder, turmeric, ginger, and chili pepper flakes. Stir in tomatoes.
3. Arrange chicken, overlapping pieces slightly, on top of tomato mixture.
4. Pour in broth and do not mix or stir.
5. Cover and cook for 6–7 hours on low.
6. Preheat oven to 200º F.
7. Carefully transfer chicken to an oven-safe plate, cover lightly, and keep warm in the oven.
8. Stir rice into the remaining liquid. Increase cooker heat setting to high; cover and cook, stirring once or twice, until rice is almost tender to bite, 30–35 minutes. Stir in shrimp, cover, and cook until shrimp are opaque in center, about 10 more minutes.
9. Meanwhile, toast almonds in a small pan over medium heat until golden brown, 5–8 minutes, stirring occasionally. Set aside.
10. To serve, season the rice mixture to taste with salt and pepper. Mound in a warm serving dish and arrange chicken on top. Sprinkle with parsley and almonds.

Nutrition:

- **Calories:** 155 g. **Fat:** 5 g. **Protein:** 56 g. **Carbs:** 45 g. **Cholesterol:** 230 mg.
- **Sugar:** 0 g.

95. Tuna and Kale

Preparation Time: 5 minutes.

Cooking Time: 20 minutes.

Servings: 4

Ingredients:

- 1-lb. tuna fillets, boneless, skinless, and cubed.
- 2 tbsps. olive oil.
- 1 cup kale, torn.
- ½ cup cherry tomatoes, cubed.
- 1 yellow onion, chopped.

Directions:

1. Heat up a pan with the oil over medium heat, add the onion and sauté for 5 minutes.
2. Add the tuna and the other ingredients, toss, cook everything for 15 minutes more, divide between plates and serve.

Nutrition:

- **Calories:** 251 g.
- **Fat:** 4 g.
- **Protein:** 56 g.
- **Carbs:** 45 g.
- **Cholesterol:** 230 mg.
- **Sugar:** 0 g.

96. Turkey With Cauliflower Couscous

Preparation Time: 20 minutes.

Cooking Time: 50 minutes.

Servings: 1

Ingredients:

- 3 oz. turkey.
- 2-oz. cauliflower.
- 2 oz. red onion.
- 1 tsp. fresh ginger.
- 1 pepper Bird's Eye.
- 1 clove of garlic.
- 3 tbsps. extra virgin olive oil.
- 2 tsps. turmeric.
- 1.3 oz. dried tomatoes.
- 0.3-oz. parsley.
- Dried sage to taste.
- 1 tbsp. capers.
- ¼ fresh lemon juice.

Directions:

1. Blend the raw cauliflower tops and cook them in a tsp. of extra virgin olive oil, garlic, red onion, chili pepper, ginger, and a tsp. of turmeric.
2. Leave to flavor on the fire for a minute, then add the chopped sun-dried tomatoes and 5 g of parsley. Season the turkey slice with a tsp. of extra virgin olive oil, the dried sage, and cook it in another tsp. of extra virgin olive oil. Once ready, season with a tbsp. of capers, ¼ of lemon juice, 5 g of parsley, a tbsp. of water and add the cauliflower.

Nutrition:

- **Calories:** 120 g.
- **Fat:** 10 g.
- **Protein:** 56 g.
- **Carbs:** 45 g.
- **Cholesterol:** 230 mg.
- **Sugar:** 0 g.

97. Baked Salmon Salad With Creamy Mint Dressing

Preparation Time: 20 minutes.

Cooking Time: 20 minutes.

Servings: 1

Ingredients:

- 1 salmon fillet.
- Mixed salad leaves.
- 2 radishes, trimmed and thinly sliced.
- 1.76 oz. young spinach leaves.
- 5 cm piece cucumber, cut into chunks.
- 1 small handful of parsley, roughly chopped.
- 2 spring onions, trimmed and sliced.

For the dressing:

- 1 tbsp. natural yogurt.
- 1 tsp. low-fat mayonnaise.
- 2 leaves mint, finely chopped.
- 1 tbsp. rice vinegar.
- Salt and freshly ground black pepper.

Directions:

1. Firstly, you heat the oven to 200º C (Gas 6).
2. Place the salmon filet on a baking tray and bake for 16–18 minutes until you have just cooked. Remove, and set aside from the oven. The salmon in the salad is equally nice and hot or cold. If your salmon has skin, cook the skin side down and remove the salmon from the skin after cooking, use a slice of fish. When cooked, it should slide away easily.
3. Mix the mayonnaise, yogurt, rice wine vinegar, mint leaves, and salt and pepper in a small dish and let it stand for at least 5 minutes for aromas to evolve.
4. Place on a serving plate the salad leaves and spinach, and top with the radishes, the cucumber, the spring onions, and the parsley. Flake the cooked salmon over the salad and sprinkle over the dressing.

Nutrition:

- **Calories:** 340 g.
- **Fat:** 30 g.
- **Protein:** 56 g.
- **Carbs:** 0 g.
- **Cholesterol:** 230 mg.
- **Sugar:** 0 g.

98. Lamb, Butternut Squash and Date Tagine

The lamb and onion's natural juices produce steam which bastes the meat as it cooks over low flame. The gentle heat keeps the inside of the tagine moist and does not dry out or burn.

Preparation Time: 15 minutes.

Cooking Time: 40 minutes.

Servings: 4 to 6

Ingredients:

- 2 tbsps. olive oil.
- 2 cm ginger, grated.
- 1 red onion, sliced.
- 3 garlic cloves, grated or crushed.
- 1 tsp. chili flake (or to taste).
- 1 cinnamon stick.
- 2 tsps. cumin seeds.
- 2 tsps. ground turmeric.
- ½ tsp. salt.
- Lamb neck fillet, cut into 2 cm chunks.
- Medjool dates, pitted and chopped.
- 14 oz. tin chopped tomatoes, plus ½ can of water.
- 14 oz. tin chickpeas, drained.
- 15.5 oz. butternut squash, cut into 1 cm cubes.
- Two tbsp. fresh coriander (plus extra for garnish).
- Buckwheat, couscous, flatbreads, or rice to serve.

Directions:

1. Preheat the oven until 140º C.
2. Sprinkle about 2 tbsps. of olive oil in a large oven-proof casserole dish or cast-iron pot. Put the sliced onion and cook on a gentle heat until the onions softened but not brown, with the lid on for about 5 minutes.
3. Add chili, cumin, cinnamon, and turmeric to the grated garlic and ginger. Remove well and cook the lid off for one more minute. If it gets too dry, add a drop of water.
4. Add pieces of lamb. In the onions and spices, stir well to coat the meat and then add salt, chopped dates, and tomatoes, plus about half a can of water (100–200ml).
5. Bring the tagine to a boil, then put the lid on and put it for 1 hour and 15 minutes in your preheated oven.
6. Add the chopped butternut squash and drained chickpeas 30 minutes before the end of the cooking time. Stir all together, bring the lid back on and go back to the oven for the remaining 30 minutes of cooking.
7. Remove from the oven when the tagine is finished and stir through the chopped coriander. Serve with couscous, buckwheat, flatbreads, or basmati rice.

Notes:

If you don't own an oven-proof casserole dish or cast-iron casserole, cook the tagine in a regular casserole until it has to go into the oven and then transfer the tagine to a regular lidded casserole dish before placing it in the oven. Add 5 minutes of cooking time to provide enough time to heat the casserole dish.

Nutrition:

- **Calories:** 404 g.
- **Fat**: 30 g.
- **Protein:** 56 g.
- **Carbs:** 30 g.
- **Cholesterol:** 230 mg.
- **Sugar:** 0 g.

99. Fragrant Asian Hotpot

Preparation Time: 15 minutes.

Cooking Time: 45 minutes.

Servings: 2

Ingredients:

- 1 tsp. tomato purée.
- 1-star anise, crushed (or ¼ tsp. ground anise).
- Small handful parsley, stalks finely chopped.
- Juice of ½ lime.
- Small handful coriander, stalks finely chopped.
- 500 ml chicken stock, fresh or made with one cube.
- ½ carrot, peeled and cut.
- Beansprouts.
- Broccoli, cut into small florets.
- 1 tbsp. good-quality miso paste.
- 3.5 oz. raw tiger prawns.
- 1.76 oz. rice noodles that are cooked according to packet instructions.
- Cooked water chestnuts, drained.
- 3.5 oz. firm tofu, chopped.
- Little Sushi ginger, chopped.

Directions:

1. In a large saucepan, put the tomato purée, star anise, parsley stalks, coriander stalks, lime juice, and chicken stock and bring to boil for 10 minutes.
2. Stir in the carrot, broccoli, prawns, tofu, noodles, and water chestnuts, and cook gently until the prawns are cooked. Take it from heat and stir in the ginger sushi and the paste miso.
3. Serve sprinkled with peregrine leaves and coriander.

Nutrition:

- **Calories:** 185 g.
- **Fat:** 30 g.
- **Protein:** 56 g.
- **Carbs:** 45 g.
- **Cholesterol:** 230 mg.
- **Sugar:** 0 g.

100. Asian King Prawn Stir Fry With Buckwheat Noodles

Preparation Time: 10 minutes.

Cooking Time: 20 minutes.

Servings: 1

Ingredients:

- 2.5 oz. shelled raw king prawns, deveined.
- 2 tsps. tamaris.
- 1.8 oz. soba (buckwheat noodles).
- 2 tsps. extra virgin olive oil.
- 1 garlic clove, finely chopped.
- 1 bird's eye chili, finely chopped.
- 1 tsp. finely chopped fresh ginger.
- 1.76 oz. celery, trimmed and sliced.
- Red onions, sliced.
- Green beans, chopped.
- 1.76 oz. kale, roughly chopped.
- Little lovage or celery leaves.
- Chicken stock.

Directions:

1. Heat a frying pan over a high flame, then cook the prawns for 2–3 minutes in 1 tsp. tamari and 1 tsp. oil. Place the prawns onto a tray. Wipe the pan out with paper from the kitchen, as you will be using it again.
2. Cook the noodles for 5–8 minutes in boiling water, or as directed on the packet. Drain and put away.
3. Meanwhile, over medium-high heat, fry the garlic, chili, and ginger, red onion, celery, beans, and kale in the remaining oil for 2–3 minutes. Add the stock and boil, then cook for 2–3 minutes until the vegetables are cooked but crunchy.
4. Add the prawns, noodles, and leaves of lovage/celery to the pan, bring back to the boil, then remove and eat.

Nutrition:

- **Calories:** 185 g.
- **Fat:** 30 g.
- **Protein:** 56 g.
- **Carbs:** 20 g.
- **Cholesterol:** 230 mg.
- **Sugar:** 0 g.

101. Prawn Arrabbiata

Preparation Time: 10 minutes.

Cooking Time: 40 minutes.

Servings: 1

Ingredients:

- Raw or cooked prawns (Ideally king prawns).
- 1.5 oz. buckwheat pasta.
- 1 tbsp. extra-virgin olive oil.

For the arrabbiata sauce:

- Red onion, finely chopped.
- 1 garlic clove, finely chopped.
- 1.2-oz. celery, finely chopped.
- 1 Bird's eye chili, finely chopped.
- 1 tsp. dried mixed herbs.
- 1 tsp. extra-virgin olive oil.
- 2 tbsps. white wine (optional).
- 14-oz. tinned chopped tomatoes.
- 1 tbsp. chopped parsley.

Directions:

1. Firstly, fry the onion, garlic, celery, and chili over medium-low heat and dry herbs in the oil for 1–2 minutes. Switch the flame to medium, then add the wine and cook for 1 minute. Add the tomatoes and leave the sauce to cook for 20–30 minutes over medium-low heat until it has a nice rich consistency. If you feel the sauce becomes too thick, add some water.
2. While the sauce is cooking, boil a pan of water, and cook the pasta as directed by the packet. Drain, toss with the olive oil when cooked to your liking, and keep in the pan until needed.
3. Add the raw prawns to the sauce and cook for another 3–4 minutes until they have turned pink and opaque, then attach the parsley and serve. If you use cooked prawns add the parsley, bring the sauce to a boil and eat.
4. Add the cooked pasta to the sauce, blend well, and then serve gently.

Nutrition:

- **Calories:** 185 g.
- **Fat:** 30 g.
- **Protein:** 56 g.
- **Carbs:** 45 g.
- **Cholesterol:** 230 mg.
- **Sugar:** 0 g.

102. Salad Skewers

Preparation Time: 10 minutes.

Cooking Time: 0 minutes.

Servings: 1

Ingredients:

- 2 wooden skewers, soaked in water for 30 minutes before use.
- 8 large black olives.
- 8 cherry tomatoes.
- 1 yellow pepper, cut into eight squares.
- ½ red onion, chopped in half and separated into eight pieces.
- 3.5-oz. (about 10cm) cucumber, cut into four slices and halved.
- 3.5 oz. feta, cut into 8 cubes.

For the dressing:

- 1 tbsp. extra-virgin olive oil.
- 1 tsp. balsamic vinegar.
- Juice of ½ lemon.
- Few leaves basil, finely chopped (or ½ tsp dried mixed herbs to replace basil and oregano).
- A right amount of salt and freshly ground black pepper.
- Few leaves oregano, finely chopped.
- ½ clove garlic, peeled and crushed.

Directions:

1. Thread each skewer in the order with salad ingredients: olive, tomato, yellow pepper, red onion, cucumber, feta, basil, olive, yellow pepper, red ointment, cucumber, feta.
2. Put all the ingredients of the dressing in a small bowl and blend well together. Pour over the spoils.

Nutrition:

- **Calories:** 315 g.
- **Fat:** 30 g.
- **Protein:** 56 g.
- **Carbs:** 45 g.
- **Cholesterol:** 230 mg.
- **Sugar:** 0 g.

103. Creamy Strawberry & Cherry Smoothie

Preparation Time: 10 minutes.

Cooking Time: 15 minutes.

Servings: 1

Ingredients:

- 3 ½ oz. strawberries.
- 3.5 oz. frozen pitted cherries.
- 1 tbsp. plain full-fat yogurt.
- 6.5 oz. unsweetened soya milk.

Directions:

1. Place the ingredients into a blender then process until smooth. Serve and enjoy.

Nutrition:

- **Calories:** 132 g.
- **Fat:** 30 g.
- **Protein:** 56 g.
- **Carbs:** 45 g.
- **Cholesterol:** 230 mg.
- **Sugar:** 0 g.

CHAPTER 14:

14 Day Meal Plan

Week 1

Days	Breakfast	Lunch	Dinner
1	Healthy chia and oats smoothie	Chicken nuggets	Garlic herb grilled chicken breast
2	Crunchy banana yogurt	Thai fish curry	Country chicken
3	Bacon and eggs with tomatoes	Fish bars	Cheesy broccoli soup
4	Cinnamon and pecan porridge	Orange and garlic shrimp	African chicken curry
5	Eggs and salsa	Garlic squash broccoli soup	Quinoa protein bars
6	Decadent cherry chocolate almond clusters	Healthy baby carrots	Artichoke petals bites
7	Bacon tacos	Bok choy samba	Pan-fried cod

Week 2

Days	Breakfast	Lunch	Dinner
1	Healthy chia and oats smoothie	Chicken nuggets	Garlic herb grilled chicken breast
2	Crunchy banana yogurt	Thai fish curry	Country chicken
3	Bacon and eggs with tomatoes	Fish bars	Cheesy broccoli soup
4	Cinnamon and pecan porridge	Orange and garlic shrimp	African chicken curry
5	Eggs and salsa	Garlic squash broccoli soup	Quinoa protein bars
6	Decadent cherry chocolate almond clusters	Healthy baby carrots	Artichoke petals bites
7	Bacon tacos	Bok choy samba	Pan-fried cod

CHAPTER 15:

FAQs

Is Intermittent Fasting Difficult to Adhere to?

It could be difficult for some people. You may experience difficulties and challenges, especially if you are still a beginner and your body still adjusts and adapts to the new routine and pattern of food intake. Once your body adapts, you will find the eating pattern more manageable and easier to follow.

The main premise is being more aware of when and what you should eat. With such awareness, you will know exactly the boundaries and limitations you have to keep in mind. Also, it would be best to pair this approach with daily exercise and making healthy food choices, like fruits, beans, veggies, healthy fats, lean proteins, and lentils.

Avoiding too much sugar and sodium is a must, too. Once your body adapts to these new guidelines, adhering to IF will no longer be that challenging.

What Is the Recommended Number of Hours/Days for Fasting?

In most cases, followers of the IF approach set their fasting window to up to 16 hours daily. Most follow this routine as it is a bit easy to adapt and adhere to. You can do it just by skipping breakfast after you ate your last meal the other day. If you can, you may also practice the IF pattern, which requires you to go without food for 24 hours straight twice every week.

Do I Still Need to Count Calories?

The answer to this will depend on the goals you want to achieve while practicing IF. It is not necessary in some cases, but if your goal is to lose weight, then you may want to still monitor your calorie intake. Also, if you plan to cut out on snacks before sleeping or go without eating for a long period, then you will notice your calorie count declining naturally. Another thing to note is that taking in foods that are mostly plant-based will also naturally lower your calorie intake.

Should Women Do IF Differently?

In most cases, men and women tend to respond differently to the IF protocol. Most women also agree that they tend to achieve better results by widening their eating window a bit. For instance, when trying to follow the 16/8 IF plan, some women noticed that they get better results after they modified the approach. That is increasing the number of eating hours to 10 and reducing the fasting hours to 14.

A wise piece of advice is to experiment and find out which one works for you. Observe the signals and cues sent by your body. Determine how it reacts to a specific IF pattern, too. Make sure to stick to an approach that seems to stimulate positive and favorable responses from your body.

Is It Safe for Pregnant or Breastfeeding Women to Fast?

Intermittent fasting is not highly recommended for pregnant women. It is mainly because your focus during pregnancy should be to supply your body with nutrients that can support your health and the growth and development of your baby. You need to eat highly nutritious foods that will help develop and build your baby's body and brain.

Also, take note that there are pregnant women who have a hard time having enough iron stores. If you do not eat the required foods every day, then it might lead to iron deficiency, which is important for your baby. Despite that, there is still no rule that bans pregnant women from practicing IF.

If you are one of those who have already practiced it and your health is at its best, then following IF is most likely safe for you. Just make sure that you only do it after receiving consent from your doctor. Also, it would be best to shorten the fasting period. If you are used to doing it for 24 hours or more, then avoid doing it while you are pregnant. You should fast for at most 14 to 16 hours only.

If you are breastfeeding, long fasting periods also need to be avoided. It is because of the constant need for your baby of nutritional milk. Fasting may have a huge impact on the quality and production of breast milk so you have to be extra careful. A wise piece of advice is to avoid fasting for more than 12 to 14 hours if you are breastfeeding to ensure that the production of milk will not be interrupted.

Make sure to observe yourself and the body, too. If you notice that your milk supply suddenly dries up and you suspect that it is because of IF, then stop fasting right away. Try to eat more regularly to find out if doing so resolves the issue. If you notice fasting greatly hampering your milk production, then maybe it is time to stop it for a while and just continue once you already stop breastfeeding.

Can I Still Work Out Even If I Am Doing IF?

Of course, you can. If your fasting period is 24 hours or more, then you may want to schedule your workouts during your non-fasting days to ensure that you have more energy to complete the sessions. You can also see other women working out even during their fasting periods, especially if their fasting takes less than 24 hours.

It is because they notice how effective exercising during a fast is in building lean muscle mass. In general, you should schedule your exercise based on how your body feels as well as the workout habits you are used to.

Conclusion

Eating on an intermittent fast can be as straightforward or as complicated as you are to choose. Some people will continue to eat healthy ahead of time and others will add another type of diet to it to see results. The ketogenic diet can work very well with this option as it limits your carbohydrates to reduce hunger and burn fat faster. However, you don't need to be on a specific diet to see results when fasting is intermittent.

The first thing to keep in mind is that you cannot eat unhealthy foods when you follow this diet type. It's good to reduce your daytime eating window to eight hours or less (or do one of the other intermittent fasting options). But if you spend that time eating desserts, fast foods, and other unhealthy foods, you will be in trouble.

First, you will not be able to lose weight if you eat this way. Fast foods and other unhealthy options are high in calories per serving, and you will likely eat more than one at a time. Even if you're eating window is smaller, you can still eat too many calories, which will halt any progress in your weight loss. Even though intermittent fasting is not about calorie intake, you should be careful not to eat too many calories. This is an aspect that can affect the effectiveness of intermittent fasting.

You will also notice that when you eat these unhealthy foods, even doing intermittent fasting, it will not improve your health. Your health will depend on a good diet rich in nutrients to stay healthy. Only fasting while eating unhealthy foods is likely to cause as many problems as you had before you started the fast.

When you eat this terrible food, you will find that you are hungry more often and find it challenging to get through your fasting periods. This is because many processed and fast foods contain chemicals and preservatives designed to make you hungry more often. If you want to see results and finish your fast without feeling hungry, now is the time to eat healthier foods.

Now, that doesn't mean you can't eat sweets or junk food sometimes. Intermittent fasting has no set rules for exactly what you're allowed to eat; you just set the hours you can eat. Eating a small cheat meal is OK, as long as you eat it during your meal times and only do it once in a while. It can be difficult at times, but eating a healthier diet will give you better results.

The trick to doing quick intermittent labor for you is to eat healthily. The more nutrients you can include in your diet, the better this fast will do for you.

The first thing to consider is to eat a lot of fruit and vegetables. Fresh produce is best because it provides many essential nutrients your body needs to stay healthy. Remember to fill your plate with fruits and vegetables at every meal to get the nutrients you need. Eating a wide variety of foods is also essential to make sure you get what your body needs without adding too many calories.

Then you need to go for good sources of protein. It would be helpful to consider going for options like lean ground beef, turkey, and chicken. Eating bacon and other fatty meats is sometimes OK; don't overdo it. Eating lots of fish will help you get the healthy fatty acids your body needs to function correctly.

Healthy sources of dairy products help you stay lean while giving your body the calcium it needs. You may have a few options like milk and yogurt (be careful with the types that have fruit and other added things as they usually have a lot of sugar), sour cream, cheese, etc. Make sure to control the salts and sugars which are not healthy for the body.

You are allowed to have carbohydrates with this diet. Carbohydrates have gotten a bad rap because many diets recommend that you avoid them.

The important thing here is to eat healthy carbohydrates for you. White bread and pasta are sugars in disguise and should be avoided. To go with whole grain and whole wheat options when it comes to carbs make sure you can get all the nutrition you need.

Eating a well-balanced diet will be the key to feeling good when you are on an intermittent fast. You can mix metals. You choose to get the best results when you do this type of fasting. You are also allowed to have a snack, as long as you are careful this happens often. If you eat junk food, you will be disappointed when you go to the scale and check that you are not losing weight. You can have treats on occasion, but make sure it's not something that diet.

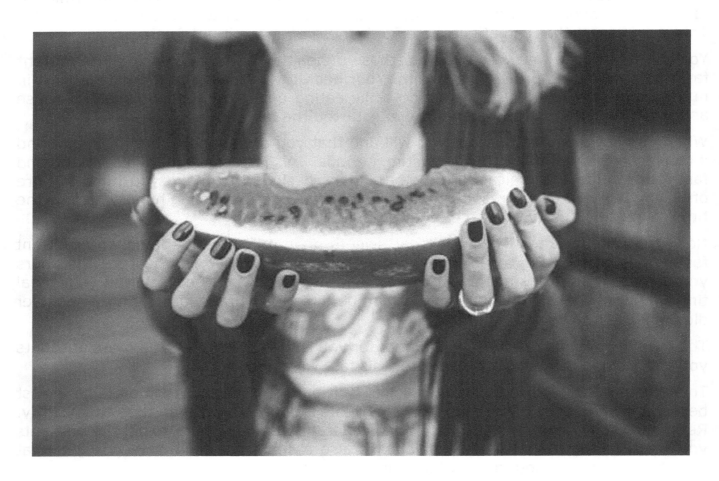